THE
THINSULIN
PROGRAM

THE
THINSULIN®
PROGRAM

THE BREAKTHROUGH SOLUTION
TO HELP YOU LOSE WEIGHT AND STAY THIN

CHARLES T. NGUYEN, MD
TU SONG-ANH NGUYEN, MD
AND MARY ANN MARSHALL

Da Capo
LIFE
LONG

Da Capo Lifelong Books
A Member of the Perseus Books Group

Copyright © 2016 by Charles T. Nguyen, MD

Set in 11.5-point Adobe Caslon Pro

Cataloging-in-Publication data for this book is available from the Library of Congress.
First Da Capo Press edition 2016
ISBN: 978-0-7382-1873-1 (hardcover)
ISBN: 978-0-7382-1874-8 (ebook)

Published by Da Capo Press
A Member of the Perseus Books Group
www.dacapopress.com

Note: The information in this book is true and complete to the best of our knowledge. This book is intended only as an informative guide for those wishing to know more about health issues. In no way is this book intended to replace, countermand, or conflict with the advice given to you by your own physician. The ultimate decision concerning care should be made between you and your doctor. We strongly recommend you follow his or her advice. Information in this book is general and is offered with no guarantees on the part of the authors or Da Capo Press. The authors and publisher disclaim all liability in connection with the use of this book.

Da Capo Press books are available at special discounts for bulk purchases in the US by corporations, institutions, and other organizations. For more information, please contact the Special Markets Department at the Perseus Books Group, 2300 Chestnut Street, Suite 200, Philadelphia, PA, 19103, or call (800) 810-4145, ext. 5000, or e-mail special.markets@perseusbooks.com.

10 9 8 7 6 5 4 3 2 1

I dedicate this book to my family. The process of writing this book took a lot of time and energy. It certainly took away time I could have spent with my four young children, Ethan, Aaron, Alyssa and Katie. I'm not sure how I can make up for missing some of your dance recitals, soccer, and baseball games. I want to especially thank my wife for believing in me. This book would only be a dream without your unwavering support.

—Charles T. Nguyen, MD

Contents

Foreword by Daniel G. Amen, MD   *ix*

Introduction: The Mind–Body Weight-Loss Connection   *xi*

PART I   GETTING STARTED

CHAPTER 1   A New Kind of Obesity Treatment:
              The Thinsulin Program   3

CHAPTER 2   Weight Loss Is a Journey, Not a Destination   11

PART II   THE SECRET OF INSULIN

CHAPTER 3   Insulin: The Powerful Weight-Loss Hormone   25

CHAPTER 4   How the Standard American Diet (SAD)
              Contributes to Obesity   35

CHAPTER 5   What Is a Carbohydrate?   43

PART III   THINSULIN PHASE ONE: THE ACTIVE PHASE

CHAPTER 6   Simple Food Choices That Help
              You Lose Weight   73

CHAPTER 7   Eat More and Still Lose Weight   89

CHAPTER 8   The Importance of Exercise   99

CHAPTER 9   Change Your Thinking   105

              Thinsulin Active Phase Milestones   *115*

PART IV THINSULIN PHASE TWO: THE PASSIVE PHASE

CHAPTER 10 Overcoming the Weight-Loss Plateau 125

CHAPTER 11 How to Eat Carbs Without Gaining Weight 133

CHAPTER 12 Exercise in the Passive Phase 147

Thinsulin Passive Phase Milestones 151

PART V STICKING WITH IT AND STAYING THIN FOR LIFE

CHAPTER 13 Staying on Track 157

CHAPTER 14 Breaking Bad Habits 167

CHAPTER 15 Controlling Food Cravings 177

CHAPTER 16 A New Beginning 183

Frequently Asked Questions 189

Appendix A: Medications for Weight Management 207

Appendix B: Weight-Loss Surgery and Thinsulin 223

Acknowledgments 233

References 235

Index 251

Foreword

As we have seen time and time again, becoming overweight can crush the body, mind, and spirit. When the pounds pack on, the mind is sent packing—thoughts become jumbled, self-confidence is shaken, and the body becomes vulnerable to a variety of illnesses.

In order to lose weight, both mind and body must join together to overcome the effects of out-of-control eating. How exciting, then, that *The Thinsulin Program: The Breakthrough Solution to Help You Lose Weight and Stay Thin* offers a scientific innovation by addressing the biological, psychological, and behavioral issues that affect your eating habits. By integrating this powerful trio, this amazing program gives you the skills to change your thinking permanently, allowing you to achieve long-term success on your weight-loss journey.

I met Dr. Charles T. Nguyen in 2004 while I was an Assistant Clinical Professor of Psychiatry and Human Behavior at the University of California, Irvine. A rising star, he had won numerous awards there as a valued professor of psychiatry. It's no surprise that Dr. Nguyen has become one of North America's leading experts on obesity as he advocates his comprehensive approach to weight management. He and his brother, Dr. Tu Song-Anh Nguyen, who provides his original weight-loss theories and medical expertise, created Thinsulin's brilliant, unique program.

This smart, forward-thinking book is backed by solid scientific research. It breaks down complex medical concepts into simple, readable explanations that teach the science behind why you choose certain foods. Thinsulin shows how you can use your body's natural rhythms to control insulin in the Active Phase to lose weight and burn fat.

Thinsulin gives you a solution to counteract the dreaded weight-loss plateau in the Passive Phase. In fact, I've never known of another program or diet that can conquer the seemingly inevitable foe of everyone trying to drop pounds. When weight loss appears to grind to a halt, dieters often become discouraged and return to the eating habits that created their weight problem in the first place.

By achieving unparalleled success in weight loss with the Thinsulin Program, you may look forward to powerful health benefits, such as reversing diabetes, high blood pressure, high cholesterol, and heart disease. Best of all, you'll find yourself enjoying heightened, enhanced health and longevity.

This accessible, stunningly simple book presents a long-term solution to a problem that costs the United States $190 billion a year. Even more important is how the Thinsulin Program supports and helps to reclaim the body, mind, and spirit of the many whose lives have become limited.

For those who struggle chronically with their weight, and others who have been unable to keep off the weight they've lost, as well as the millions who yearn to maintain their ideal weight, I highly recommend this remarkably prescient book and program.

—*Daniel G. Amen, MD*

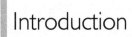 Introduction

THE MIND-BODY
WEIGHT-LOSS CONNECTION

Some of you might ask, "How is insulin related to weight loss?" In 2006, I asked that same question. Could it be that this essential hormone, which regulates blood glucose levels in the body, could also have an impact on weight? The answers amazed and moved me so much that my brother and I wrote this book in order to effectively share them with you. Here's the story behind us and behind the development of Thinsulin. (The "I" throughout this book is Dr. Charles T. Nguyen. "We" is both Dr. Charles T. Nguyen and Dr. Tu Song-Anh Nguyen.)

WHO WE ARE

Although my older brother and I are seven years apart, we share the same passion—the medical treatment of obesity. We're both doctors, and we wrote this book to help you lose weight and keep it off by sharing a powerful, effective, and simple weight-loss program.

My brother, Dr. Tu Song-Anh Nguyen, is an internist who has specialized in bariatric medicine since 1995. He earned his medical degree at Loma Linda University School of Medicine in Loma Linda, California, in 1992, and completed his Internal Medicine

Residency at UCLA Wadsworth Veterans Affairs Hospital in 1995. Since his Board Certification in Internal Medicine in 1995, Dr. Tu Song-Anh Nguyen has helped more than ten thousand patients lose weight at his three weight-loss clinics located in Santa Ana, Stanton, and Indio, California.

I took a different path from my brother. I completed my undergraduate degree in 1994, medical school training in 1998, and a psychiatry residency at UC Irvine School of Medicine in 2002. I have more than fifteen years of clinical experience treating patients with mental illnesses such as depression, schizophrenia, bipolar disorder, post-traumatic stress disorder, and similar issues.

Our childhoods prepared us to become lifelong learners. The children of Vietnamese immigrant parents, my siblings and I had humble beginnings in the United States. After the war ended in 1975, my mother raised four young children on her own while my father went to re-education camp.

In search of the American Dream, they made the brave decision to leave behind everything they knew in Vietnam and make the dangerous trek to America. My brother, Tu, left first with our father in a small wooden boat in February 1979, landing in Malaysia after five days crossing the Gulf of Thailand. They stayed in a refugee camp for nearly one year before they were sponsored to come to the United States.

I went afterward with our mother and two sisters on a small boat at the age of seven. We spent fourteen days on the raging sea with little to no food and water before we were rescued in June 1980. My little sister, who was five years old at the time, nearly died from dehydration. We stayed at a refugee camp in southern Thailand for more than three months before we were reunited with my father and brother on October 17, 1980.

Once in the United States, the six of us rented a bedroom from an elderly Vietnamese lady in Santa Ana, California. My dad came here with no money, but he was able to get a job carrying boxes at a local company in order to support our family. We didn't have much growing up. Our parents could never afford new clothes or toys for any of us. All they could give us were daily lessons that we learned at the dinner table to make the best of the opportunities America has to offer. We were driven to focus on our education.

To us, learning wasn't about memorizing a textbook. Very early on, we realized that if we understood concepts, we could apply that knowledge to all other situations. Had we only memorized math equations, for example, we wouldn't know what to do if the question deviated from what we'd memorized.

To this day, we consider learning to be vitally important. And learning never stops—it applies to all aspects of life, including how to eat. It's why, in our medical practices and in developing the Thinsulin Program, we wanted to teach our patients the science behind weight loss. Having this knowledge gives you so much more freedom.

DELVING INTO THE SCIENCE OF OBESITY

I recognized a link between psychiatry and weight loss early in my residency training in the late 1990s. Many medications used to treat schizophrenia, a mental disorder characterized by having disorganized thoughts, hallucinations, and delusions; and bipolar disorder, a mood condition that causes radical mood swings and emotional changes, also caused patients to gain a significant amount of weight, which led to increased risks for other health problems—including metabolic syndrome, high cholesterol, and diabetes. But I also noted how equally effective the medications were in managing their psychiatric symptoms and in giving my patients a chance to improve.

As their physician, I became deeply torn between the benefits of medications versus their negative side effects. I realized that while these medications might cause weight gain and metabolic effects, it would be even worse to deny my patients medications that might dampen problematic internal voices, paranoid delusions, and suicidal thoughts.

Without adequate treatment, 50 percent of patients with schizophrenia will attempt suicide; astonishingly, 16 percent will succeed. This number alone justifies the use of these lifesaving antipsychotic medications. Yet, it's far more complicated than that. Through treating thousands of patients, I saw how deeply the side effect of weight gain intrinsically damaged my already fragile patients. I felt compelled to combat this unintended effect. And so, I dedicated my medical career to managing the weight gain associated with these medications, and ultimately to helping overweight and obese people with or without mental illnesses lose weight.

I still think about my patient Natalie because she so clearly exemplifies what thousands of other patients have taught me. Natalie was a beautiful, up-and-coming ballerina deeply committed to her craft. She was just twenty years old when she was diagnosed with schizophrenia. Because Natalie refused to take her antipsychotic medication, she was treated multiple times in inpatient psychiatric hospitals. During one of her hospitalizations, I asked why she stopped taking a medication that helped to lessen the numerous voices and paranoid thoughts, and that ultimately helped her to stay out of the hospital. Natalie leaned in nervously and whispered, "Do you know how it feels to be fat? I've gained 50 pounds on this medication!"

When I put myself in her shoes, I could see how traumatic this weight gain was for her—a vital, youthful person whose weight was so interlocked with her highly coveted, wildly competitive career—and by extension, her identity. The medications distorted her carefully honed body to the point that she felt no other choice than to stop them rather than be mentally well. My consciousness radically shifted from that of a psychiatrist who saw only the importance of taking medications. I realized that the side effects put her very livelihood on the line.

I spent more than five years researching the mechanisms of weight gain to develop new ways to manage obesity associated with antipsychotic medications. In listening to thousands of patients like Natalie, I realized that medications used to help quell voices didn't just affect bodies chemically, but they also caused an unforeseen side effect: they prevented patients from feeling full. The medications increased the appetite of those who took them and made them ravenously crave more sugar and sweets.

A WIN-WIN APPROACH

After a few years, I began to alter the way I educated patients. The most effective way to teach was to keep the education simple. Focus on drinking water instead of sugary drinks; avoid cakes, cookies, ice cream, and potato chips; cut out desserts and double portions. It made sense. Initially, I called this the WIN-Nguyen, or "WIN-WIN," diet ("Nguyen" is pronounced like "Win").

The WIN-Nguyen diet addressed people's recurring cravings and increases in appetite by helping them implement healthier nutrition practices. Many patients who followed the WIN-Nguyen diet noticed a significant decrease in weight gain associated with antipsychotic medications. I published a study that showed a 55 percent reduction in weight gain by utilizing a simple, easy-to-remember strategy that patients could implement at the same time they began taking antipsychotic medications.

It's common to see two major camps in the multibillion-dollar weight loss industry: one that concentrates on exercise and physical activity, and the other that emphasizes reducing caloric intake. Personal trainers, gyms, and "boot camps" focus on the former, while weight-loss clinics focus on the latter. Patients eat prepackaged meals to reduce and control total daily calories. Nutritional shakes, often used as meal replacements, offer fewer calories as a means for weight loss. Appetite suppressants, such as phentermine, can also be used to help patients eat less, thus reducing their caloric intake. Many times, weight-loss clinics offer gimmicks like "fat burners" and vitamin B12 shots in addition to appetite suppressants, but these don't help patients lose weight. Patients can even undergo surgical interventions, such as gastric bypass or LAP-BAND® System, which will ultimately reduce caloric intake because patients are physically unable to eat as much as before. While these interventions may work for some, they are ineffective for many because they fail to address the underlying problem.

Several years later, I learned that the reduction in caloric intake doesn't tell the whole story about weight loss. I turned to my brother to learn more about the medicine and biology of weight loss. As an internist, my brother told me about the critical relationship between calories, carbohydrate intake, and one's insulin level. The hormone insulin, which lowers blood glucose, plays a key role in weight loss, as we will explain in depth in this book.

To illustrate this point, let's consider the Atkins diet. The Atkins diet consists of high protein and very few carbohydrates, and is quite effective in helping patients lose weight rapidly. But it's not reduced carbs or calories that causes weight loss. Rather, it's the effect of *lowering the body's insulin level* through a low-carb diet that is truly, biologically responsible for every patient's weight loss. That fact, however, is lost entirely on patients who've bought into the Atkins diet. Like many diets out there, it offers advice, menus, and methods to reduce your total caloric intake, but doesn't focus on why the diet works. If you know the "why" first by understanding the concepts, the "how" is a piece of cake. (Not literally!)

At first, when I heard the word "insulin," I immediately thought of diabetes. After all, it's becoming resistant to insulin's effects that leads to the development of type 2 diabetes. I told my brother that my obese patients don't have diabetes, so why should I worry about their insulin level? Dr. Tu Song-Anh Nguyen wisely took me back to my medical school years and reminded me that insulin plays a critical function in fat metabolism as well. When you lower your body's insulin level, you allow your body to burn fat and keep it from storing fat. As I got deeper into the study of insulin, I realized that the crux of every successful weight-loss program involves lowering your insulin level. Yet, rarely do these programs talk about insulin.

It's time for us to challenge the conventional weight-loss teachings and talk about a concept that is revolutionary: Weight loss isn't about eating less food or eating less fat! Simply put, weight loss is about lowering your insulin level.

A DUAL METHOD FOR WEIGHT LOSS

In 2000, my brother created a two-step program based on the insulin model called simply an "Active Passive Diet." It has helped more than ten thousand patients lose weight by lowering the insulin level (Active Diet), and to overcome the weight-loss plateau by carefully and precisely raising the insulin level (Passive Diet). Still, my brother focused chiefly on the standard medical model of weight loss by utilizing the understanding of human biology. He concentrated on foods that don't spike the insulin level, but like many obesity experts, he still primarily focused on reducing caloric intake or increasing exercise.

My brother and I had long discussions about this approach to treating obesity. What could we do to make this insulin-lowering program even more effective? We realized that what had been missing—and what we needed—was an innovative approach that also takes into account people's thoughts and behaviors. So we decided to combine our expertise and create a brand new program. Drawing from my brother's inestimable medical and bariatric knowledge to help patients lose weight by lowering their insulin levels, I bring my experience as a psychiatrist to help patients keep off the weight by addressing psychological and behavioral issues. Plenty of books tell you what to eat or how to change your behavior. But only the Thinsulin Program brings together the synergy between the working of the body and the power of the mind, representing a medical breakthrough in the management of obesity.

Any successful weight-loss program first and foremost requires you to change your way of thinking, and then to alter your eating habits. Take this simple analogy. Negative people are often miserable because of their negative thinking. So, will it work if you just tell them, "Be positive, you'll be a lot happier!" Certainly, what you said is true, but it won't help them because they haven't learned *how* to change their negative thinking through psychotherapy.

So, why would it work if your doctor tells you, "If you want to lose weight, just eat less and exercise more!" There's truth to that statement, but unless you change your way of thinking, there's a good chance that that statement won't work.

Yet, most weight-loss programs and diet plans are based on the premise of eating less and exercising more. If you stick to any of the programs, you'll lose weight initially because you're ultimately reducing your caloric intake. Similarly, a negative person might be happier by reading self-help books, doing yoga, or hanging around positive people, but unless they change the way they think through psychotherapy, their old habits will always creep back to make them miserable again. This explains why the failure rate of typical diet programs is so high. They don't utilize psychotherapy to change old ways of thinking and break ingrained bad habits.

Based on more than thirty-two years of combined medical and psychiatric expertise, we created the Thinsulin Program. It's the most effective approach to weight loss for three reasons: it uses the biological principles of how insulin works to burn fat and lose weight; the psychological principles of cognitive behavioral therapy (CBT) to change one's thinking; and behavioral modifications to break bad habits. The Thinsulin Program consists of two phases to help you lose weight, overcome the weight-loss plateau and keep off the weight for good.

Phase One, the Active Phase, involves lowering the insulin level so that your body will burn fat naturally and lose weight. After four months, you'll hit the weight-loss plateau, in which your body will no longer allow you to lose weight despite all your efforts. This is where people often get stuck using traditional weight-loss methods. The plateau occurs because your body's protective mechanism is responding to the recent weight loss by striking a natural balance, or homeostasis. In order to overcome the weight-loss plateau, you'll enter Phase Two, the Passive Phase, where you'll carefully and gently increase your insulin level. At the same time, you'll maintain your weight for another three months so that when your body allows you to lose weight again, you can return to the Active Phase to lower your insulin level.

The merger between medicine and psychiatry has created a powerfully simple and effective weight management program that teaches you to think in terms of insulin in order to lose weight and maintain it permanently. The Thinsulin Program gives you the right tools to lose weight today—and keep it off tomorrow.

PART I
GETTING STARTED

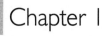

Chapter 1

A NEW KIND OF
OBESITY TREATMENT:
The Thinsulin Program

The rate of obesity in the United States continues to increase at a disconcerting pace. It's estimated that more than two-thirds of adults in the United States are overweight (33 percent) or obese (35.7 percent), equating to 78.1 million Americans. To put this in perspective, we have more overweight and obese Americans than the entire population of France (64.8 million). Since 1980, overweight and obesity prevalence among children and adolescents has almost tripled to approximately 17 percent. (*Overweight* is defined as having a Body Mass Index (BMI) between 25 and 30, and *obese* is defined as a BMI over 30.)

At the same time, the stigma of obesity is stronger today than it was forty years ago. An astonishing study by the Rudd Center for Food Policy and Obesity at Yale University assessed people's attitudes toward obesity. Rather than be overweight, 4 percent would rather be blind, and 5 percent would rather lose a limb. Between 15 and 30 percent also said they would rather be depressed, become an alcoholic, give up the possibility of having children, and walk away from their marriage than be obese. Nearly half said they would rather give up a year of their lives than be fat.

For many years, obese people have been treated unfairly, and obesity has been viewed as a result of consistently poor lifestyle choices. But recent evidence now implicates hormonal and metabolic processes in the development and progression of obesity. In 2009, Dr. Louis Aronne, an internationally recognized expert in the field, published that obesity meets all the criteria for a medical disease, including a known cause, recognized signs and symptoms, and a range of structural changes. Obesity is caused by many different factors, involving genetics, physiology, and behavior. In 2011, for the first time in medical history, the American Association of Clinical Endocrinologists (AACE) declared obesity as a disease state.

Two years later, the nation's largest medical association, the American Medical Association (AMA), adopted a policy that recognizes obesity as a disease requiring a range of medical interventions. At the AMA House of Delegates 2013, they passed Resolution 420, stating that, "The ramifications of obesity warrant a paradigm shift in the way the medical community tackles this complicated issue."

Yes, there must be a sea change when it comes to weight loss. To say the current way isn't working is more than an understatement. How many times have you heard doctors tell patients to "eat less and exercise more"? If only it was that simple, we would be a thin nation! We would also have fewer life-threatening diseases—cancer, heart disease, high blood pressure, and diabetes—that are related to obesity.

Each year, approximately forty-five million Americans go on a diet and spend nearly $33 billion on commercial weight-loss programs and products. Too many promise miracles, but ultimately fail to deliver. While a small subset of people may benefit from them, there are many, many more who don't achieve long-term weight loss. Multiple research studies have shown that 95 to 98 percent of people who lose weight gain it back within five years. Only 2 to 5 percent succeed in keeping off their weight. A recent study published in the *American Journal of Public Health* reported that, in any given year, the average obese woman and man have about a 1 in 124 and 1 in 200 chance, respectively, of returning back to a normal weight.

Some consumers opt for the next pill, product, or gimmick that promises easy weight loss without dieting or exercise. These are the ones who are most often disappointed when they don't lose what they think is the "right" amount of weight or any weight at all, leading to devastating blows to their self-esteem. With repeated failures, they continue to choose methods that are either unproven or over-hyped. They believe they have very few choices.

In treating more than thirteen thousand patients at our weight-loss clinics in Southern California, we realize again and again how difficult it is for people to be in this predicament. They want to lose weight, and yet don't know how to do it successfully. So, they rely on stories they've heard, like the close friend who dropped a quick ten pounds on a fad diet; or the sister who dropped two dress sizes by cutting out fat; or the stories on a late-night infomercial for diet pill supplements—willing to follow any diet plan, however misguided, that they believe might work.

But there is a better way. People are hungry for something different. We see it in their eyes when they enter our clinics, and that hunger changes to relief and hope when they hear success stories about the Thinsulin Program.

FINALLY THIN

Christina, a forty-eight-year-old store manager, came to our Lor-phen Medical weight-loss clinic in Riverside, California, in 2011 after trying numerous programs without success. She told us that she noticed from day one how different this weight-loss program was. Rather than focusing on reducing caloric intake through replacement shakes, the Thinsulin Program taught Christina to change her thinking, break her bad eating habits, and open her mind to the fact that insulin level is at the core of weight loss. After three months, she lost 49 pounds! She has been able to keep off the weight for the past two years, and believes it's blue skies ahead. Christina shared, "I never knew in all those years of dieting how simple losing weight really is. I thought it was about weighing food and prepackaged meals and starving. I didn't know I could eat so often, wherever I wanted, feel so liberated, and lose weight at the same time."

Our method works because it addresses the *root* of the problem. In medicine, you can patch up a wound, slow the bleeding, or perform a countless number of stopgap measures to fix a problem temporarily, but without finding the root cause, that problem will continue to occur. Simply put, if you understand the "why" first by learning the concepts of how insulin affects the body, the "how" of weight control is easier.

As you read on, you'll learn that insulin is the magic hormone that is the key to help you lose weight and inches permanently. When you reduce your caloric intake, you'll lose weight, but when you lower your insulin level, you'll burn fat. Thinsulin, a new term that combines three words—think, thin, and insulin—teaches you to think in terms of insulin rather than in terms of calories.

Fernando, twenty-three, is 6 feet tall and weighed 293 pounds with a BMI of 39.7 when he started the Thinsulin Program. He had recently married his high school sweetheart, so he wanted to get back on track toward being healthy again. During his junior year, he had been a muscular 215 pounds, and had played team football as a nose guard. These days, with his hectic work schedule and living off fast food, he'd gained more than 75 pounds four years after graduating from high school.

Within the first week of following the Thinsulin Program, Fernando lost 10 pounds, an amount of weight loss that's very common. He was amazed to see his weight drop every week, even though he was eating five times per day. He was extremely happy to lose 30 pounds after four weeks without having to starve himself, drink any shakes, or eat any prepackaged meals. He even did it while eating at his usual fast food restaurants, simply by changing the way

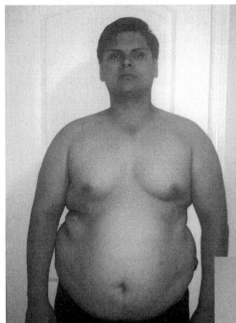

Fernando Before:
September 2013, 293 pounds

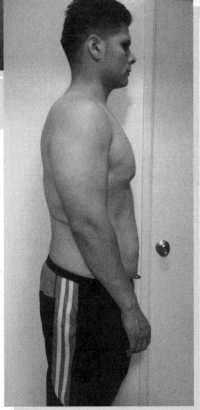

Fernando After:
January 2014, 219 pounds

he thought about food. Instead of counting calories, he thought in terms of insulin, and he chose foods that didn't spike his insulin level. When he ordered hamburgers, he ate more meat and avoided the buns and fries. He ate more green vegetables, which kept him full while keeping his insulin level low. At Mexican restaurants, instead of eating tamales, he ate chicken fajitas with salsa. "I didn't think it would be this easy!" he shared excitedly. "I never felt hungry."

The Thinsulin Program taught Fernando how to break his old eating habits. He was shocked to see how much fat he was able to lose around his stomach area. His clothes were loose and he could fit into his old jeans again. Feeling motivated, Fernando hit the gym and began to lift weights. He continued to weigh in every two weeks. Eight weeks later, he weighed 242 pounds, losing a total of 51 pounds.

He continued to work out three times a week. Friends, coworkers, and family members noticed how much weight he was losing and began to ask questions. He told them that he was learning about Thinsulin, a two-step program that was teaching him how to lose weight first and then overcome the weight-loss plateau afterward by thinking in terms of insulin and not calories. He had lost weight before, but said, "I have never lost so much fat in my life." He dropped an additional 11 pounds at the end of three months, weighing in at 231 pounds.

Entering his fourth month on the Thinsulin Program, Fernando continued to lose weight, but not at the same amazing rate as during the first three months. He expected this. He knew that his body was fighting the weight loss as he approached the weight-loss plateau. He was excited to shift gears soon and learn the second step of the program in order to overcome the plateau. As Fernando reflected back on his four-month journey, he noticed that the way he thought about food and his eating habits had changed completely. The Thinsulin Program had given him the knowledge and skills to help him lose weight and keep it off.

For the first time in his life, he felt confident that he would win his struggle against obesity. At the end of four months, he weighed 219 pounds, representing a total of 74 pounds or a whopping 25.3

percent weight loss (see Figure on page 7). His BMI decreased from 39.7 to 29.7, going from being morbidly obese to overweight.

Put that weight loss in perspective for a moment. Imagine if you lost a quarter of your current weight in four months without having to starve, drink shakes, or eat replacement meals? Would you be happy with that result? As you can see from the pictures, Fernando's belly fat was reduced tremendously when he took steps to lower his insulin level. Imagine how you would look if you burned off that much belly fat? It *is* possible with the Thinsulin Program, especially if you're seeking a solution to the endless cycle of dieting and weight fluctuations.

Insulin is what *truly* makes other diets like Atkins, Paleo, and South Beach all work behind the scenes. Underneath the hype, if those plans succeed, it's by lowering your insulin level. But these plans omit something crucial—an important system grounded in research and clinical experience to help you change your thinking, change your eating habits, and ultimately, change your eating behavior. That's what makes Thinsulin different! This is the missing link that the Thinsulin Program provides. Thinsulin offers a medical breakthrough by uniquely harnessing the working of the body and the power of the mind to manage obesity.

THE THINSULIN PROGRAM

The Thinsulin Program is not another gimmick. It will work for you. The results speak for themselves. At The Obesity Society's 31st Annual Scientific Meeting Poster Session during ObesityWeek 2013, the Thinsulin Program captured attention by demonstrating a weight loss of 10.8 percent, or 23 pounds, over an average of eighty-six days.

Twenty-three pounds may not seem that significant as you're reading it now. I want you to stop reading for a moment and pick up a twenty-five-pound dumbbell, a two-year-old child, or a nineteen-inch flat-screen TV. Try carrying it while you're reading this chapter. You'll realize fairly quickly how heavy twenty-three pounds actually is. Can you imagine how much lighter and freer you would feel if you lost this much weight?

The significance of a 10.8 percent weight loss cannot be understated. Studies have shown that even modest amounts of weight loss, just five to ten percent of body weight, can result in significant improvements in obesity-related diseases, such as type 2 diabetes, coronary artery disease, stroke, high blood pressure, high cholesterol, obstructive sleep apnea, abnormal menses, infertility, and certain types of cancer.

Maya Angelou once said, "When you know better, you do better." After reading this book, you'll certainly know your mind better, and your body will be recharged and ready to do better. You'll have the right skills to find long-term success in your ongoing weight-loss journey.

Chapter 2

WEIGHT LOSS IS A JOURNEY, NOT A DESTINATION

This journey begins with the power of a simple decision. Today is the day that you choose to be healthy by losing excess weight. When you prepare to lose weight, you might not ponder what it takes to make lifestyle changes over time. Rather, you set goals to lose a certain amount of weight by a certain date. You'll wake up early to go to the gym. You'll stay on course by restricting what you eat. You want to get to your goal weight so badly!

Unfortunately, life is never that simple. Getting from point A to point B isn't always as the crow flies. Possibly, your boss will give you extra work, leaving you without enough time to cook dinner. Or, in your quest to lose weight, life might throw you a curveball in the form of an injury, leaving you unable to exercise for several months, just as you're starting the Passive Phase. Does that mean you give up? Not at all. This is why you must see weight loss as a journey rather than a destination.

Setting a goal to lose a certain amount of weight is similar to traveling to a certain destination. Once you get to your destination or goal of weight loss, where do you go from there? What do you do next? Do you keep walking the same path? That's the major problem with dieting and why it leads to so much failure. Too often, negative, all-or-nothing thinking traps people in unrealistic standards of being perfect. The thinking goes, if you mess up once, you might as well give in to your cravings and eat whatever you want. You set the bar so high that it's impossible to make any significant changes in your eating habits. So you continue doing what you're most comfortable doing, and revert back to your old ways. The monstrous cycle continues.

If you see weight loss as a journey, one little mistake won't be so catastrophic. It can serve as a meaningful lesson to enrich your personal growth. You might have your ups and downs, but you'll learn from these examples to find success down the road. Seeing weight loss as a journey allows you to take the small steps necessary to make the changes in your life. It's much less intimidating than taking one giant leap.

————

Jennifer, forty-six, is a successful business owner. She prides herself in working hard and it shows in the success of her home-health business. While she enjoys this success, her inability to lose weight and keep it off represented an unspoken or unconscious failure. This failure weighed on her heavily.

No matter which weight-loss programs she enrolled in, she was unable to keep the weight off. Even if she came close to her goal, she would regain most of it fairly quickly due to the normal stress of raising two children along with running a busy practice. "I thought dieting was starving myself," Jennifer said. She viewed weight loss as a destination, rather than a journey. Once she made her goal weight, she didn't know what to do next. She realized she needed to change her way of thinking if she wanted to stop her weight from "yo-yoing" up and down.

In September 2014, Jennifer's hairstylist told her about Lorphen Medical. At 5'5" and weighing 193.2 pounds, she was committed to lose weight again. Jennifer realized that this was the right program after the first visit. The concept of insulin made sense to her, especially given her medical background as a registered nurse. She

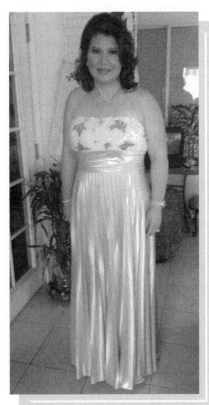

Jennifer Before:
September 2014, 193.2 pounds

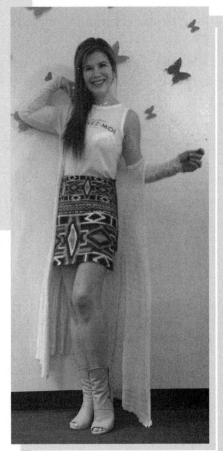

Jennifer After:
August 2015, 139.2 pounds

had spent years educating her patients with diabetes on how to eat better. She finally made the connection between insulin and weight loss. Thinking in terms of insulin helped her choose the types of food that would allow her body to burn fat. In addition, she liked the fact that Thinsulin isn't a diet, but a program that was built upon the principles of biology, psychology, and behavioral therapy to walk her through her journey.

Now that Jennifer has lost 54 pounds, her self-perception as a failure has turned around completely. In September 2015, she celebrated a year of keeping the weight off. She is happy that her most recent doctor's visit showed an improvement in her cholesterol and fasting sugar. More important, she feels more confident in herself and it shows in her life.

"Losing weight really opened up a lot of doors," Jennifer said. "I feel much more confident about myself."

OVERCOMING COMMON MYTHS

As with every successful journey, you'll need to ask yourself why you want to lose weight. Are you doing this just so that you can fit into your swimsuit? Or, do you want to be healthier so that you can enjoy your golden years?

People have different motivations for weight loss. One study showed that dieting driven by health concerns leads to fewer medical problems than dieting driven by motivation to change physical appearance. People with the latter tend to engage in more extreme dieting strategies, including using laxatives, avoiding meals, and excluding food groups.

Still, appearance is a very powerful motivator and can evoke strong emotions, and we're more likely to be attracted to the physical aspects of weight loss. There's nothing wrong with wanting to be able to fit in jeans without a muffin top spilling over, or, for guys, to feel comfortable taking off your shirt again.

In the end, it's not so much what the motivation is. It's your *willingness to change* that's the most important factor in this journey.

As you follow the guidelines of the Thinsulin Program, it may be hard initially to go against what you've been taught for many years. Comedian W.C. Fields once said, "A dead fish can float downstream, but it takes a live one to swim upstream."

As you embrace your weight-loss journey, you may encounter challenges. Your willingness to change, to swim against the current, will help you resist the temptations and clear the cognitive distortions, or distorted thinking. We'll go over several common cognitive distortions that you might encounter throughout your journey so that you can be prepared to overcome them.

Myth #1: "I'm on a diet."

Dieting evokes painful memories of suffering and deprivation. From past experience, you might remember how you need to prepare yourself mentally for a serious round of dieting. You might binge on sweets or carbs before starting on this ordeal. Or you might put it off until after the holidays or birthdays so that you don't have to suffer too much during times of celebration.

When you're on a diet, you might typically restrict your caloric intake to the point where your stomach is growling. You fight the hunger pangs by drinking more water, hoping that it will make you feel full. If you do well, you reward yourself, only to feel guilty afterward. You then proceed to punish yourself—and the no-win situation continues.

We need to break this endless loop by changing your thinking. With Thinsulin, you don't starve yourself. You can eat as much as you want to. Throughout both the Active and Passive Phases, you eat a full five times a day. For lunch and dinner, you must have at *least* a portion of proteins and a portion of green, leafy vegetables. You can have more if you want, just as long as you're feeling satisfied and full. You're not starving with Thinsulin because it *isn't* a diet. It's a program that teaches you to think in terms of insulin.

Kelly, a twenty-four-year-old student, tried the Thinsulin Program after failing several popular diet programs. "I quickly learned how this wasn't a diet. I can eat as much as I want, unlike before, when I was starving myself (which made me gain even more weight). Overall, I dropped three sizes!"

It's important for you to avoid using the word *diet* altogether. When you lose weight during the Active Phase, friends, coworkers, and family members will notice and ask which diet plan you're on. Tell them you're *not* on a diet. If you even utter the word *diet*, then you're still unconsciously operating in a diet mentality. You're only setting yourself up for the whole monstrous cycle of punishment and reward. You must break free of the old way of thinking.

By avoiding the word *diet*, you're removing the deprivation, suffering, and punishment that come along with dieting. Instead, let your friends know that you're in the Active Phase and you're lowering your insulin level. They may reply, "Say what? Active Phase? Insulin?"

You go on to say, "My goal is to lower my insulin level so that my body can burn rather than store fat. I'm thinking in terms of insulin, so I'm selecting foods or drinks that won't increase my insulin level."

On the Thinsulin Program, you'll choose foods for yourself, rather than being forced to follow a prescribed meal plan with recipes. When you're in the Passive Phase, you'll learn how to reintroduce carbs and sweets into your meals without causing weight gain. Even during this phase, though, it's still important for you to avoid using the word *diet*.

Myth #2: "I don't have time to eat."

For the first few months, the excitement of a new program will often keep you on track. Over time, you might find that your old ways and thinking will seep back into your life and sabotage your progress. On some days, you find yourself too busy to eat breakfast or lunch because your schedule doesn't permit you the time to eat. You're too busy to make sure you fulfill all your responsibilities to everyone else but yourself. But how is that fair? Aren't you just as important? The answer is yes!

Take a moment and think back to all the times you've skipped meals. Ask yourself why? Were you too busy with your children's activities? Is your job taking away from your time to eat? Do you simply not have the time to eat? We hear this quite often as an excuse to skip meals.

If you continue to neglect yourself and abuse your body by skipping meals and not eating properly, your body will fail one day. Then, it doesn't matter how much you want to help others—because you won't be able to physically help them. *You have a responsibility to yourself because you're that important!* You're important enough to give yourself fifteen minutes out of your busy schedule to ensure that you'll eat your five meals.

We're not asking for much. It's not like you're completely selfish and ignore your other responsibilities. All we're asking you to do is take fifteen minutes out of your day to plan for what you're going to eat the next day.

On the Thinsulin Program, you can decide to cook or go to a restaurant. But you must plan. This is no different than anything else you do in life. If you manage a store, do you need to plan ahead of time to be successful? You need to plan to see who's going to work a certain shift. You plan for your work. You plan for your vacation. You just don't decide to show up for a camping trip without planning ahead of time. You plan what you're going to pack, what you're going to eat, and which freeway you're taking.

Fifteen minutes. Look at your schedule. Plan how you're going to fit your meals into your schedule. Make sure you do this throughout the Active and Passive Phases.

So the next time you say, "I don't have time to eat," stop and challenge this distortional thinking! You *do* have time to eat. You simply didn't leave any time for yourself to plan ahead. Remember, you're just as important as your job, family, or friends. Your health has to be a priority as well. Please don't forget this as you go through your journey.

Myth #3: "I've been doing well. It's OK to
cheat because this one time won't matter."

As you experience the Active Phase, you'll face many temptations. Unfortunately, it's not just coming from commercials or billboards encouraging you to indulge in those fries. It's often coming from the people you love. They might offer you a slice of cake or some home-made lasagna. They might tell you, "Come on. Loosen up a little. Have a bite." They don't do it out of spite, they do it out of love because they want you to enjoy life. They don't quite understand the concept of insulin.

To many of your friends and loved ones, they still operate in the realm of thinking eating fewer calories is okay. In this mindset, eating a little of something won't matter that much because you're still minimizing the calories. But this is faulty. As you operate on the concept of Thinsulin, you'll be thinking in terms of what will spike your insulin level. Even a little bit of sweets, grains, or starchy vegetables can do this. It's not so much the quantity, but the ability of the foods to spike insulin that matters most.

It's very important to challenge this cognitive distortion. Cheating *does* matter, and as you read on about how insulin works in the body, you'll see why.

It's important to avoid cheating even when you're staying on track. When you're seeing success, it's common to ease up and be complacent. We sometimes see this with our patients, who stop eating their morning fruit as a snack. They slowly deviate from the program, doing what they find to be most convenient for them. It happens. It's just human nature. Unfortunately, when a bump in the road occurs, you may not be ready to face the problem because you're unprepared. This puts you at risk for cheating. For example, let's take college athletes trying to adjust to professional sports. The fame of success might make players more complacent, so they don't train as hard. Their performance suffers simply because they deviated from their regular training that got them to that competitive level.

If you're staying on track during the Active Phase, don't get complacent! Continue to build upon your success and challenge yourself to stay focused. The longer you're able to continue, the more this will become a way of life for you. The routine will help establish a new habit that will help you not to overeat during the Passive Phase.

Myth #4: "I've blown it for the day already, so what's the point of continuing?"

This is the typical mindset of a dieter with all-or-nothing thinking. This negative thinking traps the dieter into being either impeccable or worthless. It doesn't have to be that black or white. With unrealistic expectations of being perfect, one little mistake can be seen as a complete letdown, making it more difficult to pick up where you've left off.

Everyone makes mistakes, and chances are that you may, too. That's OK! Challenge this negative thinking immediately. Just remember, a mistake in a journey is an opportunity to learn. If you mess up, try to understand why you ate that candy bar. Was it because you didn't eat lunch? Make corrections for next time and move on. Do your best to stay on track and don't just give up.

Jesse, a construction worker and father of two, was ecstatic that he dropped 70 pounds as a result of his Active Phase. As he entered the Passive Phase, he was allotted the usual half a portion of carbs a day before returning in two weeks for a weigh-in. He didn't return until six months later. He had regained 40 pounds and desperately wanted to go back on the program.

He shared that many friends and family members congratulated him after he lost all that weight. He was proud of his achievement, but soon the success got the best of him. He became complacent as he slowly deviated from the program. Instead of seeing this as a journey, Jesse didn't take the time to learn about how the Passive Phase works to maintain weight loss. Over time, he found himself skipping lunch and snacking on more nuts. Then, it was ice cream and crackers. Soon he was overdoing it on mashed potatoes and fried chicken, and drinking sodas again. As he continued to share, Jesse became a bit defensive and said, "I know I messed up. I thought I could control myself after being on a diet that long."

As you can see from this example, just the fact that Jesse used the word *diet* means that his old way of thinking had seeped back into his life. The faulty thinking of dieting takes him back to being caught in the monstrous cycle of punishment, reward, and guilt. Furthermore, when Jesse ate more junk foods, he felt horrible for messing up. "So I kept on eating because I thought it was no use since I already cheated."

You might have these moments in your life where you'll feel like a failure. Don't get caught in all-or-nothing thinking! Failure is when you don't pick yourself up and go back to the program. Jesse didn't fail because he came back to learn. This was merely a bump in the road, or a setback for Jesse, but certainly not a failure.

It's easy for anyone to fall off the wagon. If this happens, rather than beat yourself up, understand that there are still things to learn. In the case of Jesse, he thought that once he reached his weight-loss goal, he was done. He didn't have a chance to learn what to do in the Passive Phase to keep it off.

Myth #5: "I don't need to eat for enjoyment."

Let's address an important psychological barrier that sabotages most dieters. They often justify their restrictions through the idea that they "eat to live, *not* live to eat." Unfortunately, that phrase is unattainable. It simply goes against your basic instincts of enjoyment. You can't deny your body of enjoyment. And who wants to, anyway? You need the enjoyment that life has to offer, especially if your life is filled with stress. You look forward to that long vacation on a sandy beach or to that girls' night out. Certainly, enjoying your food will be a part of this picture.

Everywhere you look, advertisements reinforce the basic fact that you need to enjoy life. You see images of happy people dancing and singing while drinking a soda. Or you see pictures of a juicy burger and fries seemingly screaming out from the television to eat them. So to deny the fact that enjoyment can't be part of your life will only set you up for failure. Eventually, that restrictive thinking, "eat to live, not live to eat" will turn into "I live to eat, not eat to live." When you're not prepared to address the enjoyment aspect, you're more likely to give in to the hedonistic urge and eat whatever and whenever you want.

Tania is a forty-four-year-old homemaker with a spiky crown of red hair. She shared that she had lost 20 pounds in the past by drinking a replacement shake for both breakfast and lunch. After a few months, she got sick of drinking the shakes. She craved some hearty food to chew on. She missed going out to restaurants or eating with her family at dinnertime. To her, what's life without enjoying her food?

"In the end, the weight loss wasn't worth starving myself with those darn shakes," she said. "My body was screaming out for comfort food."

At the same time, you can't just eat whatever you want, anytime you want, and expect to keep the weight off. There must be a balance between your hedonistic drive and your control over what you eat. How do you find this balance? *Change your thinking.*

Let's examine this further. Say this statement out loud: "I enjoy eating." If you enjoy eating, then you should be able to feed that enjoyment and eat whatever you want and whenever you want. It gives your hedonistic drive the green light to commit the sin of gluttony. We're exaggerating this point a bit, but you get the picture. In the end, you still haven't struck a balance between enjoyment and control.

Let's take the same statement and switch the order of the two words, "enjoy" and "eating." Now, say this out loud: "I eat for enjoyment." Is it a bit awkward to say? That's expected because you've never been taught to say this. Look at how powerful the new statement is. You can still enjoy what you eat, but it's more controlled. The sentence, "I eat for enjoyment," instead of "I enjoy eating," emphasizes control first over enjoyment. Once you reach the Passive Phase, you can have your "enjoyment food" such as pasta or ice cream *after* you've eaten your vegetables and proteins.

By changing your thinking to acknowledge enjoyment while still having control, your way of thinking will be more in line with reality. You no longer have to view food as your enemy. It's not! You're not restricted to suffering by eating bland food or drinking shakes for the rest of your life. This isn't another diet where you have to deprive yourself. You'll be eating five times a day and feeling full. And once you hit the weight-loss plateau, you'll be able to have more of your favorite foods again in the Passive Phase. When you get to the Passive Phase, it's important for you to constantly remind yourself of this statement, "I eat for enjoyment." The enjoyment food typically increases your insulin level and includes sweets, grains, starchy vegetables, or high-glycemic fruits. You'll see.

Throughout your weight loss journey, you'll encounter good as well as bad days. Celebrate your successes and allow them to continue to motivate you. If distortional thinking sabotages your success, rather than throwing in the towel, it's important to take a step back to see what went wrong, then try again. Take small steps and you'll see how the Thinsulin Program can help change your thinking and behavior.

PART II
THE SECRET OF INSULIN

Chapter 3

INSULIN:
The Powerful Weight-Loss Hormone

op nutritional experts point to consuming excessive carbohydrates as the culprit to obesity and, subsequently, to chronic diseases such as hypertension, type 2 diabetes, and heart disease. On average, Americans eat about 250 to 300 grams of carbohydrates per day, accounting for about 55 percent of their caloric intake.

Insulin is one of the most important hormones in the human body, and your diet—including your carb intake—is key when it comes to regulating your insulin level. For the most part, people tend to associate insulin with diabetes. You might know people who need to inject themselves with insulin or have an insulin pump to bring down their blood glucose (blood sugar). But even if you don't have diabetes, insulin still plays a critical role in your weight. Here's how.

THE RIGHT BLOOD GLUCOSE LEVEL
KEEPS YOUR CELLS ALIVE

We as human beings require energy to survive. Our cells store energy in the form of a compound called adenosine triphosphate, or ATP.

Cells need glucose to create ATP, and without ATP, they will eventually die. Unlike plants that make glucose through a process called photosynthesis, we can't create our own glucose, so we rely on our diets. Everything we eat will eventually be converted to glucose for the cells to use in order to power our body to function.

If our blood glucose level is too low, not enough glucose will travel to our tissues and organs, leaving our cells unable to generate enough ATP to function. On the other hand, too much glucose in the blood will impede blood flow. You can see what happens when you add too much sugar to water. The water doesn't flow very well. (Thus you hear the saying, "slow as molasses.") If blood doesn't flow well due to a high glucose level, it won't be able to deliver the necessary oxygen to the cells, leading to cell deaths over time. This is why uncontrolled diabetes might lead to blindness and kidney failure—too much glucose blocks the flow of oxygen to the cells. As you can see, it's important for the body to maintain a certain blood glucose level, where there's not too much or too little glucose.

INSULIN: REGULATING YOUR BLOOD GLUCOSE LEVEL

Every time we eat, a sudden shot of glucose enters our bloodstream after the food is digested in the stomach. Our body needs to adjust quickly so that the blood glucose can be delivered to the cells for use. What regulates the blood glucose? The answer is insulin, a hormone produced by the beta cells in the pancreas. Our body releases insulin right before and during eating, so that insulin can signal the liver, muscle, and fat tissues to take glucose out of the blood (thus lowering the blood glucose level). Insulin binds to the insulin receptors in the muscle cells, signaling the cells to absorb the glucose from the bloodstream and store it as glycogen. As the blood glucose level drops, the insulin release slows or stops. To protect the body from blood glucose getting too low (known as hypoglycemia or low blood sugar), another hormone, glucagon, stimulates cells to break down glycogen and release glucose. And so, a balance is maintained.

To prepare the body for a sudden flood of glucose after a meal, our bodies begin to release insulin before we take a bite of food. Isn't that amazing? Our body produces insulin by the mere smell or sight of food. The sweeter the brain believes the meal will be, the more it will tell the pancreas to produce insulin, even before the food enters our mouth.

Let's say you're eating a candy bar. As you eat it, the food is broken down in the stomach and absorbed as glucose into your bloodstream. Your body responds by increasing its secretion of insulin. Within a few minutes, there's been a dramatic rise in insulin level—known as the first phase—in order to bring down the glucose level in your blood as quickly as possible.

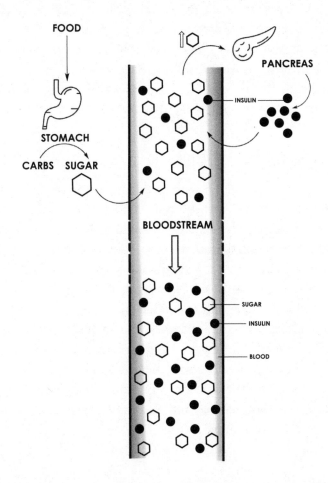

In addition, the more you ate in the previous meal before your candy bar, the more insulin will be released from storage this time. However, if the blood glucose level remains high, the beta cells will produce and release more insulin in pulses every ten to twenty minutes until the blood glucose returns to normal levels.

Besides the pancreas, the brain also produces its own supply of insulin. The brain needs a lot of fuel to run properly, so it also needs to regulate blood sugar levels. Insulin in the brain is thought to enhance learning and memory.

Stress can also affect your blood glucose level. The stress hormone noradrenaline (aka norepinephrine)—known as the fight-or-flight response—inhibits insulin release because the body needs to store extra blood glucose to reach the muscle cells in order avoid danger. For example, say you need to flee from a robber. You want enough blood glucose in reserve so that your body has ample energy to escape danger. You don't want insulin released to lower your blood glucose. You might blame comfort food for weight gain when you're stressed out, but stress itself, along with sweets, also increases insulin.

INSULIN DEFICIENCIES AND DISEASE

Diabetes is often associated with problems in the insulin pathway. There are two kinds of diabetes: Type 1 diabetes is caused by a lack of insulin production by the pancreas. Type 2 diabetes is caused when insulin is present, but the cell receptors are resistant to its effects, which results in high, unregulated blood sugar levels. Poorly managed diabetes might eventually lead to organ damage such as blindness, amputations, infections, and kidney failure.

Type 1 diabetes, which accounts for 10 percent of all cases, often affects younger children who are born with a condition where their own immune system destroys the insulin-producing cells in the pancreas, leading to little or no insulin production. As a result, their bodies don't store food as fat, and also burn any existing fat. These children are often very thin.

On the other hand, type 2 diabetes is often seen in adults who are obese. Unlike type 1, where the body doesn't produce insulin at all, type 2 diabetes is caused by having high insulin levels for too long. Remember, insulin is meant to be a fast-acting hormone, with its primary job being to bring down blood glucose. If you're eating too many carbs or on a high-sugar diet, your insulin levels will remain high all the time. Over time, the insulin receptors become desensitized to insulin and won't work as well.

Here's an example. Imagine insulin as a key and the cells' insulin receptors as a lock. If you use the key frequently to open the lock, eventually the lock gets worn down from overuse and doesn't work as well. As a result, you might need to try more keys to find the right match to open the lock.

The same can be said with type 2 diabetes. The more carbohydrates and sweets you eat, the more insulin the pancreas has to produce. Over time, the excessive insulin wears down the cells' insulin receptors, leading to insulin resistance. In order for insulin to successfully bind to the insulin receptors, the pancreas has to produce more of it. Then, like anything else that is overworked, the pancreas begins to break down and doesn't function correctly to produce insulin. In this case, people with type 2 diabetes might need to inject themselves with insulin in order to control the blood glucose.

When you develop insulin resistance, the ability of your brain cells to absorb sugar decreases, thus reducing brain function, leading to an increased risk of developing mild cognitive impairment (MCI), a condition in which people experience more memory problems than are usually present in normal aging and in dementia. In fact, people with type 2 diabetes are at least twice as likely to develop Alzheimer's, a condition that's projected to affect ten million baby boomers in their lifetimes. Many people with diabetes have brain changes that are hallmarks of both Alzheimer's disease and vascular dementia.

While it's unclear if diabetes actually causes Alzheimer's, they both have the same root: an overconsumption of carbs, especially sugar, which affects insulin. A study published in the *Journal of Alzheimer's*

Disease followed 937 elderly people (median age of 79.5 years) over several years to see if an association between calories consumed and incidences of mild cognitive impairment (MCI) or dementia existed. The study found that the risk of MCI or dementia was elevated in subjects who ate more carbs, but was reduced in subjects who ate more fat and more protein. In other words, a dietary pattern of consuming lots of calories from carbs, and relatively few from fat and proteins, might increase the risk of MCI or dementia in elderly people.

Another report, by Dr. Jose Luchsinger from Columbia University College of Physicians and Surgeons, in New York, NY, reported that hyperinsulinemia, a consequence of higher adiposity or fat and insulin resistance, is also related to a higher risk of dementia, including late-onset Alzheimer's disease.

INSULIN AND WEIGHT MANAGEMENT

In the past, you might not have associated insulin with weight management, but you need to. Remember, what you eat will affect how much insulin your body will produce. The more carbohydrates and sweets you eat, the more your body will produce insulin, leading to insulin resistance over time.

You may notice that your friends who are thin seem to eat a lot of foods without gaining weight. On the other hand, friends who are obese seem to gain weight despite eating less. The difference between your friends is their insulin levels. Your obese friends may have a condition called *hyperinsulinemia*, or a state of high insulin levels, while your thin friends may have normal to low insulin levels. However, your thin friends won't continue to stay thin if they overload their bodies daily with extra amounts of high-glycemic-index (GI) carbohydrates. Their insulin receptors will become desensitized, leading to insulin resistance. At that point, they will gain more weight by storing fat.

The answer lies in how insulin affects different cell types. When insulin binds to the insulin receptors of brain, muscle, and liver cells, it promotes glucose absorption and storage as glycogen. The brain, muscle, and liver have a limit on how much glycogen they can store. Once these storages are full, the body still has to remove the excess glucose from the blood and put it somewhere. Therefore, insulin binds to the insulin receptors of fat cells, signaling the fat cells to absorb the excess glucose into the fat cells and store it as fat. In addition, insulin tells the fat cells to take in fatty acids from the bloodstream, turn them into fat molecules, and store them as fat droplets. In short, insulin causes the body to store fat either by taking in extra glucose or fatty acids in what's called "adipose tissue," usually around your belly, hips, and thighs.

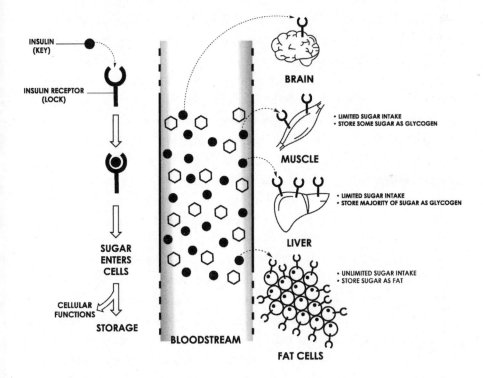

At the same time, the high insulin levels prevent your body from using fats for fuel, leaving you unable to burn fat. You're adding more fat, but you can't burn it off. In addition, elevated insulin levels hinder your body from breaking down glycogen to glucose in case your blood glucose drops. Because your body isn't able to burn fat or break down glycogen for energy to power your cells, your body will make you crave carbohydrates, especially sweets, in order to get the needed sugar. Unfortunately, the moment you grab that donut or cookie, the extra sugar will be converted to fat, and your insulin levels will rise even higher. As this cycle continues, your pants won't fit over time, with high insulin levels as the culprit.

But the opposite occurs when you lower your insulin level. Your body won't store any fat and it will also burn fat, leading to weight loss. The best way to lower your insulin level is to eat fewer carbs such as breads, pasta, and sweets. As your blood glucose drops because of decreased intake of carbs, your body doesn't need to produce as much insulin. Remember, the amount of insulin your body will produce depends on what you ate for your last meal. If your most recent meal didn't require much insulin release, your pancreas won't have to produce as much insulin this time around in the first phase of insulin release. So, if you continually eat foods that don't require much insulin release, your pancreas will produce less insulin over time.

Your fasting insulin (insulin level measured at a fasting state) doesn't drop immediately. It still takes time for your body to lower your fasting insulin level. In a study published in 1970, it showed that, during fasting, the insulin level dropped to its lowest in about five days. However, if you're not fasting but just eating fewer carbs, this process takes a bit longer. It may take as long as *three weeks* to see a drop in your insulin level.

How exactly does lowering your insulin level lead to weight loss? When you're eating fewer carbs and your body doesn't need to produce as much insulin, your brain and muscle cells still need glucose for energy. Because your cells aren't getting the glucose from what you're eating, this forces the fat cells to release fatty acids into the bloodstream, which will be converted to ketone bodies. The ketone bodies are used by the brain and muscle as an alternate fuel to glucose. There's no need to store fat because the body needs to burn fat to use as energy. As you can see, your body burns fat, not stores it, when your fasting insulin drops.

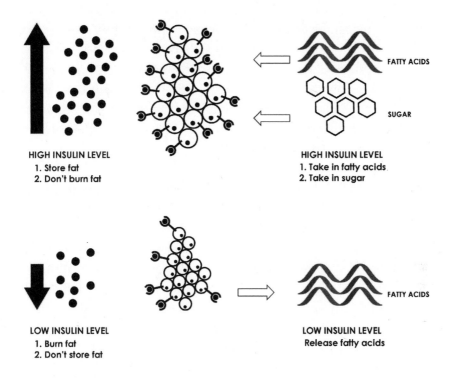

HIGH INSULIN LEVEL
1. Store fat
2. Don't burn fat

FATTY ACIDS

SUGAR

HIGH INSULIN LEVEL
1. Take in fatty acids
2. Take in sugar

LOW INSULIN LEVEL
1. Burn fat
2. Don't store fat

FATTY ACIDS

LOW INSULIN LEVEL
Release fatty acids

WHEN YOU "CHEAT" ON A DIET

What happens if you've done well keeping your fasting insulin level low, but you decide to cheat with some sweets? Let's go through this example in more detail. Let's say the sweet in question is a piece of apple pie.

The pancreas already produces insulin at the sight and smell of the pie as it anticipates you eating it. As soon as you put that piece of pie in your mouth, your blood glucose will rise, and the beta cells in the pancreas will produce insulin. Typically, insulin that was kept in storage while your blood sugar level was normal will be released all at once, peaking within minutes, to bring down the blood sugar. However, because you've been lowering your intake of carbs and sweets, your pancreas didn't have to produce as much insulin, so there's not a lot left in storage. There might not be enough insulin to bring down the blood glucose level, so your body will stimulate the beta cells to produce and release insulin in pulses every ten to twenty minutes until the blood glucose level returns to a normal level. Consequently, the beta cells produce extra insulin for storage as the body prepares for the next meal. As you can see, your insulin level now is higher than before you cheated with that piece of pie. When this occurs, your body will revert back to storing fat and won't burn fat. Remember how long it takes for your body to lower your fasting insulin level? Yep, it takes up to *three weeks*.

Cheating—even with the lowest-calorie cookies you can think of —is probably the biggest reason why people on diet programs fail. The cookies might only contain 30 calories each, but if they have high sugar content, they will increase your insulin level, causing your body to store fat again for three weeks. That's a pretty dramatic consequence for a simple slip, but we're here to tell you the truth, not to sugarcoat it (no pun intended) or promise results that the body simply can't deliver. What we can tell you with great certainty is that if you *don't* cheat, your fasting insulin *will* lower, and you *will* lose weight!

The bottom line is, insulin is a vital hormone that's involved in glucose regulation as well as fat storage in the body. If you increase your insulin level, you can expect to gain weight and increase fat. Thinsulin helps you lower your insulin level, so you'll lose weight and inches.

Chapter 4

HOW THE STANDARD AMERICAN DIET (SAD) CONTRIBUTES TO OBESITY

In our medical practice, we've noticed that a greater percentage of our second-generation Asian patients, for example, are overweight or obese and have greater risks for diabetes than those of the first generation. Basically, our patients who have spent more time eating traditional American foods suffer more health-wise.

Maricel is a twenty-six-year-old nurse who strolled into our clinic straight from work wearing dark blue nursing scrubs. At 4'10", she weighed 192 pounds, which placed her squarely in the obesity category with a higher-end BMI of 40.1. Maricel's jet black hair matched that of her mother's, who accompanied her to our office. Her mother, Emily, was born in the Philippines, but Maricel grew up in the United States eating typical Western foods. Maricel told us she preferred snacking on French fries along with cookies and chips, and drinking sodas, milkshakes, and juices, while her mother hasn't adopted the American diet. It was difficult to see a young, vibrant woman suffering from high blood pressure and type 2 diabetes that were likely caused by obesity. We believe her health issues have a lot to do with eating the Standard American Diet. (How ironic is that abbreviation? SAD, but true.) Maricel's story is not unique. There are approximately two hundred fifty thousand fast food restaurants in the United States, and over a twenty-year period, our total fast food consumption has risen from 2 percent to 10 percent of total energy intake per person.

That said, SAD foods are also increasingly being consumed in other parts of the world. Prior to the growth of fast food chains in Asian countries, for example, obesity wasn't nearly as prevalent there as it is now. According to the Overseas Development Institute report, the number of overweight and obese adults in the developing world has increased nearly four times to approximately one billion since 1980. So it's not surprising to see an explosion of diabetes worldwide. The rate of diabetes and the upsurge of fast food chains in those countries is no coincidence. Over many generations, Asian people have adapted to a higher intake of carbohydrates, like rice noodles, found in their traditional diets, but their bodies are unable to handle the massive overload of carbs, and especially sugar, that are found in SAD fast foods and desserts. What does that tell us? Too much blood glucose and too much insulin!

Let's take a typical fried chicken meal. Many people see fried food as a main culprit for weight gain. We agree that high-calorie fried food isn't the healthiest food, but it's actually the rise in insulin it causes that leads to the weight gain. For example, fried chicken is often breaded, and these carbs increase insulin. Oftentimes, a fried chicken meal is accompanied by coleslaw, mashed potatoes, biscuits topped with honey, and, of course, a soda.

Let's put aside the total number of calories for a second. Let's look at the typical fried chicken meal through a different lens—in terms of its effect on insulin. Chicken is breaded before being fried. Bread increases the insulin level. Mashed potatoes: besides the starch, the gravy is often sweetened with high-fructose corn syrup (HFCS)—an added sugar. The coleslaw is definitely sweetened with sugar as well as HFCS. Biscuits are made of flour and have a high glycemic index. That *definitely* increases insulin level! And finally, without a doubt, sweets such as honey and sodas will spike your insulin level. It's all about insulin, insulin, insulin! That's why the rates of obesity and diabetes have exploded and become a world-wide epidemic.

TOO MANY CALORIES FROM SUGAR

Although food that causes too much insulin is a big culprit in the obesity problem, many people—even medical professionals and organizations—still believe obesity is mainly an issue of consuming too many calories, and that it doesn't matter if the calories came from carbs, fats, sugars, or proteins. You've undoubtedly heard the phrase, "Calories *in* equal calories *out*." (A calorie is defined as a unit of heat energy.) According to the Centers for Disease Control and Prevention (CDC), "A calorie is a calorie regardless of its source." And numerous weight-loss apps track your calories to help you lose weight.

On the surface, this seems to be true. In fact, we've operated on this train of thought for many years. But when you challenge this thinking for a second, you'll find that the "calories in, calories out" concept is drastically oversimplified. Eating too many calories does contribute to weight gain, but that's not the whole story. There's no way that the calories from a 4-ounce chicken breast are the same as the calories from a can of sugar-filled soda! You learned in the previous chapter about the effects of sugar on insulin, so you know that the effect of eating sugar isn't the same as eating protein.

We don't want you to think that sugar is all bad—our bodies need sugar, such as glucose, as an energy source to power the body's cells. What we have to worry about is *too much* sugar. Like anything in life, moderation is the key. Consider this interesting fact: our hunter-gatherer ancestors ten thousand years ago consumed about 20 teaspoons *a year* of sugar. A typical 20-ounce soda or sports drink contains about 17 teaspoons of sugar *per drink*. How many sports drinks have some of us reveled in after a particularly difficult workout? If you only drank one, that's almost the equivalent of what our ancestors had in one year.

The United Nations (UN) and the World Health Organization (WHO) have recommended that sugar should account for no more than 10 percent of daily calories. If an average person eats 2,000 calories per day, only 200 of those calories should come from sugar. That would translate to about 8 teaspoons of sugar per day. But how much are we actually eating per day?

It's estimated an American consumes about 140 pounds of sugar per year. That's twenty-eight 5-pound bags of sugar or about 30 teaspoons of sugar per day. That's almost four times more than what is recommended by the UN and the WHO. Compared with what our ancestors used ten thousand years ago, Americans today consume almost five hundred fifty times more. WOW! Now consider all the other carbs you're eating on top of this, and you can see why we're experiencing an outright obesity epidemic.

How is it possible to eat that much sugar in one year? It would be very difficult to eat twenty-eight 5-pound bags of pure sugar. The sugar surely must be hidden in something that makes it easy for us to consume that much of the stuff annually without really noticing.

In the standard American diet, the obvious culprits would be sugary beverages and junk food. When you exclude naturally occurring sugars like fructose in fruits, the major source of added sugar is soft drinks. According to the USDA, it's estimated that 33 percent of all added sugars consumed come from soft drinks, 10 percent from sweetened fruit drinks, 5 percent from candy and cake, and 4 percent from morning cereals.

You'll be surprised to know that many prepared foods and low-fat products are big contributors to the sugar problem as well. Prepared foods like canned vegetables and fruits, condiments, and peanut butter account for 26 percent of the added sugars. You've been taught to think that low-fat products are good for you. The truth is the opposite! Low-fat products actually contain *a lot* of sugar to make up for the lack of taste. Check the label to see how much sugar is in low-fat salad dressing.

LOW-FAT DIETS DON'T WORK

Some experts hypothesize that the association between low-fat diets and obesity can be traced back to the 1970s. In 1977, the US government recommended a decrease in dietary fat intake to no more than 30 percent of calories while *increasing carbohydrate intake* from 55 to 60 percent of calories. Since then, we've certainly seen an increase in carbohydrate intake. According to the National Health and Nutrition Examination Surveys (NHANES), total caloric excess from carbohydrates greatly increased, while total fat intake slightly decreased from 1974 to 2000. Is it a mere coincidence or is there some correlation with cutting down fat intake and increasing carbohydrate intake to a rising obesity rate? We might not know for sure, but we do know this: recent research shows that low-fat diets failed to show improvement in obesity rates or long-term cardiovascular outcomes. If this is the case, low-fat diets aren't effective for weight loss due to their high-sugar content.

While low-carb diets restrict the sugar content, they typically don't restrict saturated fat intake. Again, common sense would tell us that too much of anything would not be good for us. Would foods high in saturated fat lead to more heart attacks? Supporters of low-carb diets don't think so, as they have cited research evidence supporting the health benefits of low-carb diets. These studies, however, didn't follow the participants for a decent length of time—only six months or less. When these studies are longer in duration (at least twelve months or longer), there's no clear cardiovascular benefit to low-carb diets over other diets.

Unlike both low-fat and low-carb diets, Thinsulin takes into consideration the amount of carb and saturated fat intake. We heed the nation's top nutrition advisory panel recommendations to cut down on large servings of *saturated fats* such as fatty meats, fried foods, whole milk, and butter in order to reduce the risks for cardiovascular disease. Notice that the warning is for saturated fats—*not* for cholesterol. In 2015, the same panel reversed close to forty years of government warnings on the consumption of cholesterol in a diet that may include eggs, shrimp, and lobster. For this reason, you're able to eat shellfish with Thinsulin because shellfish don't spike insulin level, and cholesterol is no longer considered a "nutrient of concern."

YOU DON'T NEED TO GIVE UP ALL CARBS

So, which diets work for weight loss? More than sixteen published trials show the effectiveness of low-carb diets in weight loss by severely restricting carbohydrate intake such as starches and sugar. Over time, this indeed lowers the insulin level, allowing the body to burn rather than store fat.

But it's not necessary to restrict all carbohydrates because not all carbohydrates are the same. Some carbs spike insulin, while others don't. What matters is that you eat foods that won't increase your insulin. In the next chapter, you'll learn more about these foods.

Obesity is more than just a calories problem. On the surface, it might seem like the reason fast foods and sugary drinks are to blame for weight gain is their high calories, but beneath, it's the increased insulin level these foods create that directly impacts obesity.

Roni, fifty-nine, is married with two grown children in their thirties. She looks forward to retirement next year when she turns sixty. She has battled obesity since the fifth grade. Her weight has fluctuated ever since. She believes the obesity problem lies with the way weight loss is taught. "The food pyramid that we learn is upside down," Roni shared. "I gained so much weight eating the food groups of that pyramid."

Twelve years ago, she weighed her lifetime heaviest at 197 pounds. She lost 22 pounds by eating less and choosing healthier foods, but she was stuck at 175 pounds for a year. She came to Lorphen Medical Clinic, in Riverside, California, to overcome this plateau. Within eight months, she lost 50 pounds, bringing her weight down to a trim and healthy 125 pounds. For the first time in her life, she has been able to maintain that weight for over a year. She found that the Thinsulin Program gave her more choices and

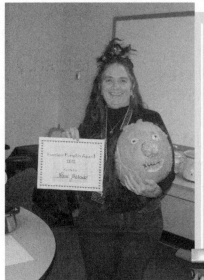

Roni Before:
October 2013, 175 pounds

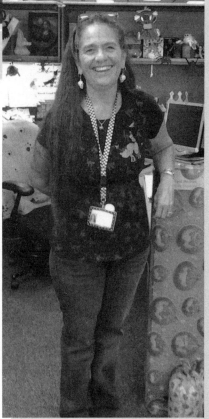

Roni After:
October 2014, 124 pounds

freedom. "I can't do a weight-loss program that makes you eat a certain way," Roni said.

As she looks forward to retirement, she knows that Thinsulin will be a part of her life. She doesn't want to go back to her old ways of thinking in terms of calories. She sees her food as a source of enjoyment. Most important, she sees the foods in terms of insulin.

Chapter 5

WHAT IS A CARBOHYDRATE?

While on the Thinsulin Program, you'll reduce the amount of carbohydrates you consume, and instead, consume more proteins and fiber. Carbohydrates, also known as starches or sugar, provide the body with energy, but many of them also cause an increase in the body's insulin level—some dramatically so! In this chapter, we'll clarify what on earth a carbohydrate really is, so that we're all on the same wavelength.

A carbohydrate is a molecule that consists of carbon (C), hydrogen (H), and oxygen (O). A carbohydrate can be in the form of monosaccharides, disaccharides, or polysaccharides.

Monosaccharides include glucose (universal sugar), fructose (sweet sugar), and galactose (milk sugar). (All three monosaccharides have the same number of carbon [6], hydrogen [12], and oxygen [6] atoms, but they have different chemical arrangements.)

All-powerful *glucose* is known as "universal sugar" because it's the energy of life. Every single organism on the planet needs it to survive. Plants and trees produce glucose in a process known as photosynthesis, where carbon dioxide (CO_2) is combined with water (H_2O) using light energy. Every single organism metabolizes glucose for energy and gives off carbon dioxide and water, which are recycled again by plants to make more glucose.

Fructose is what sweetens our fruits. It's also found in honey. Fructose is 1.73 times sweeter than table sugar, sucrose.

Galactose is found in milk and whey. It's less sweet than fructose and glucose. Nursing infants obtain the galactose required for their development from mother's milk. The body needs galactose for different functions, such as keeping the immune system healthy.

Disaccharides are two units of monosaccharides bonded chemically to each other. Examples include table sugar sucrose and lactose or milk. Sucrose consists of glucose and fructose, while lactose consists of glucose and galactose.

Polysaccharides are super long molecules containing thousands of glucose hexagon rings joined to each either by *alpha bonds* to form starch or glycogen, or *beta bonds* to form cellulose or fiber. Humans have enzymes only to break down alpha bonds, not beta bonds. That's why humans can't digest fiber. We'll focus first on complex carbohydrates such as starch and glycogen.

STARCH AND GLYCOGEN

Starch is a polysaccharide, a complex carbohydrate. It's usually stored in fruits, grains (rice, pasta, bread, or corn), or in potatoes. Glycogen is the analogue of starch. While starch is a chain of glucose made by plants, glycogen is a chain of the same glucose made by animals. Our body converts the extra glucose from foods into glycogen for storage in the liver and muscle cells.

Starch is easily digested into individual glucose because most organisms, including humans, possess enzymes to break down alpha bonds. The heat from cooking also helps to break down the alpha bonds. That's why your glucose level rises faster when you eat well-cooked rather than uncooked starches. For example, cooked carrots will increase your blood glucose level more rapidly than compared with raw carrots because the cooking heat breaks down those bonds that hold the glucose chain together. The quick rise in glucose level would stimulate your beta cells in the pancreas to produce insulin.

When starch is refined and processed, it's usually well cooked and grinded. Grinding foods helps to break up the alpha bonds too, so that's why eating processed foods will spike your insulin more than eating whole foods. For example, according to a study published in the *American Journal of Clinical Nutrition*, cooking ground rice causes a higher level of insulin responses compared with whole rice.

Starch is classified as *rapidly available, slowly available, or resistant,* depending on how quickly it's broken down into individual glucose.

1. *Rapidly available* starch breaks down quickly into glucose, making it high on the Glycemic Index (GI). (How quickly the glucose level rises after a particular food is digested is referred to as "GI," as we'll discuss in the next section.) It includes refined and processed foods such as white rice, white bread, and breakfast cereals.
2. *Slowly available* starch breaks down gradually, so it's considered a medium GI. Grains, whole wheat, and some fruits such as bananas and pineapple are considered slowly available starch.
3. *Resistant* starch is defined as any starch that isn't fully digested in the small intestine, therefore, its GI is low. It includes seeds, legumes, and unprocessed whole grains.

You've been taught to believe that eating processed foods is worse than eating whole foods. Yes, there's a lot of truth in that, but you have to realize that even whole starches will spike insulin. The key question we always need to ask and answer is, "Will this food spike my insulin level?" Processed foods may spike it quicker than whole foods, but the end result is the same. That's why, during the Active Phase of weight loss, you don't ever want to eat processed or whole starches. However, during the Passive Phase, when you're gradually increasing your insulin level while maintaining your weight, you may consume starches. Whole foods would be better choices than processed foods.

What carbohydrates you eat, and how much, can impact your insulin release. Different carbohydrates contain different amounts of monosaccharides. Glucose is more likely to stimulate the pancreas to release insulin. More insulin is released when there's a higher level of glucose. Therefore, measuring how quickly glucose would rise in your blood will help determine which carbohydrates will be best for you to eat to minimize spiking your insulin level.

GLYCEMIC INDEX

Glycemic Index (GI) measures how carbohydrates react in your blood. GI is a ranking system (0 to 100 score) that classifies foods based on how quickly they raise blood sugar level. An example of a food with a high GI is pure sugar, which has a GI of 100. Foods with a high GI are digested and broken down very rapidly, causing a quick rise in blood sugar, and subsequently, the insulin level. Any food with a high GI will raise your blood sugar level. Remember that rapidly available starch such as refined and processed starch has a high GI.

Carbohydrates with a low GI tend to be digested, broken down, and absorbed slower, leading to a gradual rise in blood sugar and subsequent insulin level. An example of a food with a low GI is almonds, which have a GI of zero. Foods with a low GI won't impact your blood sugar levels. These types of foods make you feel fuller, and give you more energy. Make these foods your friend. They might limit your weight gain and could even lead to weight loss.

Again, foods are classified as low, medium, or high GI. Medium and high-GI foods will rapidly increase our insulin level, while low-GI foods are less likely to do so.

High-GI Foods = GI of 70 or more
Medium-GI Foods = GI of 55 to 69
Low-GI Foods = GI of 0 to 54

Because GI is calculated on a per-carbohydrate basis, it doesn't tell the whole story. For example, two foods that have the same GI might have a different effect on blood glucose if one has a higher carbohydrate content than the other. The effect of a carbohydrate's content or serving on blood glucose is known as *Glycemic Load (GL)*. You can calculate the Glycemic Load (GL) of a particular food by multiplying that food's ranking on the GI by the carbohydrate content (weight in grams in a single serving), then dividing the total by one hundred. This, no doubt, sounds complicated, but the point is that you need to consider the content and portion—as well as the GI—of any foods. Luckily, you don't need to do any math, as the GL is usually listed below in the chart! A GL of 10 or less is considered low, while a GL of 20 or more is considered high. (Just like the GI, you'll want to go for a lower number.)

The GI value alone cannot accurately predict what your actual blood sugar will be. The only way to get a fuller picture is to actually measure your blood sugar responses to foods. This is why you can't solely use the GI as a replacement for measuring your blood sugar if you have diabetes. This concept, however, is worth understanding so that you can make better choices. Below is a chart that details the different types of foods:

GLYCEMIC INDEX AND GLYCEMIC LOAD FOR 100+ FOODS

Glycemic index and glycemic load offer information about how foods affect blood sugar and insulin. The lower a food's glycemic index or glycemic load, the less it affects blood sugar and insulin levels. Here is a list of the glycemic index and glycemic load for more than 100 common foods.

FOOD	Glycemic index (glucose = 100)	Serving size (grams)	Glycemic load per serving
BAKERY PRODUCTS AND BREADS			
Banana cake, made with sugar	47	60	14
Banana cake, made without sugar	55	60	12
Sponge cake, plain	46	63	17

continues

continued

FOOD	Glycemic index (glucose = 100)	Serving size (grams)	Glycemic load per serving
Vanilla cake made from packet mix with vanilla frosting (Betty Crocker)	42	111	24
Apple, made with sugar	44	60	13
Apple, made without sugar	48	60	9
Waffles, Aunt Jemima (Quaker Oats)	76	35	10
Bagel, white, frozen	72	70	25
Baguette, white, plain	95	30	15
Coarse barley bread, 75–80% kernels, average	34	30	7
Hamburger bun	61	30	9
Kaiser roll	73	30	12
Pumpernickel bread	56	30	7
50% cracked wheat kernel bread	58	30	12
White wheat flour bread	71	30	10
Wonderbread, average	73	30	10
Whole wheat bread, average	71	30	9
100% Whole Grain bread (Natural Ovens)	51	30	7
Pita bread, white	68	30	10
Corn tortilla	52	50	12
Wheat tortilla	30	50	8
BEVERAGES			
Coca Cola®, average	63	250 mL	16
Fanta®, orange soft drink	68	250 mL	23
Lucozade®, original (sparkling glucose drink)	95±10	250 mL	40
Apple juice, unsweetened, average	44	250 mL	30
Cranberry juice cocktail (Ocean Spray®)	68	250 mL	24

continues

continued

FOOD	Glycemic index (glucose = 100)	Serving size (grams)	Glycemic load per serving
Gatorade	78	250 mL	12
Orange juice, unsweetened	50	250 mL	12
Tomato juice, canned	38	250 mL	4
BREAKFAST CEREALS AND RELATED PRODUCTS			
All-Bran, average	55	30	12
Coco Pops, average	77	30	20
Cornflakes, average	93	30	23
Cream of Wheat (Nabisco)	66	250	17
Cream of Wheat, Instant (Nabisco)	74	250	22
Grapenuts, average	75	30	16
Muesli, average	66	30	16
Oatmeal, average	55	250	13
Instant oatmeal, average	83	250	30
Puffed wheat, average	80	30	17
Raisin Bran (Kellogg's)	61	30	12
Special K (Kellogg's)	69	30	14
GRAINS			
Pearled barley, average	28	150	12
Sweet corn on the cob, average	60	150	20
Couscous, average	65	150	9
Quinoa	53	150	13
White rice, average	89	150	43
Quick cooking white basmati	67	150	28
Brown rice, average	50	150	16
Converted, white rice (Uncle Ben's®)	38	150	14
Whole wheat kernels, average	30	50	11
Bulgur, average	48	150	12

continues

continued

FOOD	Glycemic index (glucose = 100)	Serving size (grams)	Glycemic load per serving
COOKIES AND CRACKERS			
Graham crackers	74	25	14
Vanilla wafers	77	25	14
Shortbread	64	25	10
Rice cakes, average	82	25	17
Rye crisps, average	64	25	11
Soda crackers	74	25	12
DAIRY PRODUCTS AND ALTERNATIVES			
Ice cream, regular	57	50	6
Ice cream, premium	38	50	3
Milk, full fat	41	250 mL	5
Milk, skim	32	250 mL	4
Reduced-fat yogurt with fruit, average	33	200	11
FRUITS			
Apple, average	39	120	6
Banana, ripe	62	120	16
Dates, dried	42	60	18
Grapefruit	25	120	3
Grapes, average	59	120	11
Orange, average	40	120	4
Peach, average	42	120	5
Peach, canned in light syrup	40	120	5
Pear, average	38	120	4
Pear, canned in pear juice	43	120	5
Prunes, pitted	29	60	10
Raisins	64	60	28
Watermelon	72	120	4
BEANS AND NUTS			
Baked beans, average	40	150	6

continues

continued

FOOD	Glycemic index (glucose = 100)	Serving size (grams)	Glycemic load per serving
Blackeye peas, average	33	150	10
Black beans	30	150	7
Chickpeas, average	10	150	3
Chickpeas, canned in brine	38	150	9
Navy beans, average	31	150	9
Kidney beans, average	29	150	7
Lentils, average	29	150	5
Soy beans, average	15	150	1
Cashews, salted	27	50	3
Peanuts, average	7	50	0
PASTA and NOODLES			
Fettucini, average	32	180	15
Macaroni, average	47	180	23
Macaroni and Cheese (Kraft)	64	180	32
Spaghetti, white, boiled, average	46	180	22
Spaghetti, white, boiled 20 min, average	58	180	26
Spaghetti, wholemeal, boiled, average	42	180	17
SNACK FOODS			
Corn chips, plain, salted, average	42	50	11
Fruit Roll-Ups®	99	30	24
M & M's, peanut	33	30	6
Microwave popcorn, plain, average	55	20	6
Potato chips, average	51	50	12
Pretzels, oven-baked	83	30	16
Snickers Bar®	51	60	18

continues

continued

FOOD	Glycemic index (glucose = 100)	Serving size (grams)	Glycemic load per serving
VEGETABLES			
Green peas, average	51	80	4
Carrots, average	35	80	2
Parsnips	52	80	4
Baked russet potato, average	111	150	33
Boiled white potato, average	82	150	21
Instant mashed potato, average	87	150	17
Sweet potato, average	70	150	22
Yam, average	54	150	20
MISCELLANEOUS			
Hummus (chickpea salad dip)	6	30	0
Chicken nuggets, frozen, reheated in microwave oven 5 min	46	100	7
Pizza, plain baked dough, served with parmesan cheese and tomato sauce	80	100	22
Pizza, Super Supreme (Pizza Hut)	36	100	9
Honey, average	61	25	12
The complete list of the glycemic index and glycemic load for more than 1,000 foods can be found in the article "International tables of glycemic index and glycemic load values: 2008" by Fiona S. Atkinson, Kaye Foster-Powell, and Jennie C. Brand-Miller in the December 2008 issue of *Diabetes Care*, Vol. 31, number 12, pages 2281-2283			

Let's put this concept into practice. If you look at GI only, you'll see that a white bagel (GI of 72) and whole-wheat bread (GI of 71) have almost the same GI. Will eating either one of them cause the same insulin release? We know you got this one right. While both will cause your insulin to spike, the white bagel will cause more of an increase in your sugar and insulin level than the whole-wheat bread because of the difference in GL (25 to 9).

We sometimes group carbohydrates together as one, although there are three different types (monosaccharide, disaccharide, and polysaccharide). Each type can cause different responses to insulin. You can measure the insulin response by looking at the GI. High-GI foods will cause the blood glucose level to rise, triggering an increase in insulin level, which, in turn, will promote fat storage. The opposite is true with low-GI foods, which is important in the Active Phase. When you transition to the Passive Phase, you may have foods that raise your insulin. However, you don't want to overdo it, so still consider low-GI and low-GL carbohydrates such as whole grain and brown rice.

FIBER

Cellulose is also a polysaccharide that consists of thousands of the same glucose linked together, but unlike glycogen and starch, it's linked by beta bonds. Cellulose is very tough—it's used to build the cell walls and most of the supporting structures of green plants. Humans don't have the enzyme to break down the beta bonds. So when we eat the cellulose or *fiber* of green, leafy vegetables and plants, we can't digest it. However, ruminants such as cows and horses, along with termites, bear enzymes to digest the beta bonds so they can obtain energy from grasses and wood.

There are two main types of fiber: soluble and insoluble. Soluble fiber dissolves in water, while insoluble fiber doesn't. Americans on average eat more insoluble than soluble fiber.

Soluble fiber, found in flaxseed, fruits, and vegetables, becomes gel-like in water, thus, helps to hydrate stool. This allows it to slip through the intestines smoothly, reducing constipation. In addition, soluble fiber can reduce appetite and increase satiety.

Because fiber is not fully digested and it's dissolvable in water, the foods turn thick and slurry, thus slowing down absorption in the small intestine. As a result, you feel fuller, and you might eat less. A study published in the *American Journal of Clinical Nutrition* showed that food intake reduced by 11 percent by adding one kind of soluble fiber to a diet.

Since fruits and vegetables dissolve in water but aren't fully digested, they are readily fermented in the gut to produce short-chain fatty acids and prebiotics, which may have many health benefits in weight management. *Prebiotics* promote the growth of normal bacteria living inside the colon by providing nutrients. Approximately one hundred trillion bacteria, which is ten times the number of total cells in the adult human body, are colonized inside the human intestine. Undigested fruits and vegetables provide food on which the bacteria thrive. Using up the glucose from the fiber would lower the insulin level, thus leading to weight loss. We know that these gut bacteria even help to maintain a healthy body weight in children.

Short-chain fatty acids produced by soluble fiber have been shown to improve mineral and nutrient absorption, strengthen our immune system, and even reduce the risk of colon cancer.

Insoluble fiber provides the mass or bulk for forming stool. This allows for the solid but soft stool to move easily through the GI tract. Insoluble fibers include kale, spinach, nuts, seeds, bran, and whole-grain foods. Consider amaranth, kamut, millet, and quinoa that contain high levels of fiber as alternatives to wheat. These insoluble fibers are great choices for the Passive Phase, but *not* the Active Phase because they can still spike insulin levels due to the GI and GL. For example, quinoa has a GI of 53, so it will still spike your insulin. The best insoluble fibers that have a GI and GL of zero are green leafy vegetables such as kale and spinach.

The next time someone mentions carbohydrates, you'll know instantly that not all carbohydrates are created equally. Don't just stop there! Try to visualize what happens to your insulin level if you eat those carbs. Imagine the bathroom scale going up if you eat high-GI foods, or foods that increase your insulin, and the scale going down when you eat low-GI foods, or foods that lower your insulin. Your most important job is to think in terms of insulin. Always!

THE TRUTH ABOUT FRUCTOSE AND HIGH-FRUCTOSE CORN SYRUP

The food industry and nutritional experts are locked in a furious debate over the effects of fructose on health. The food industry cites the fact that fructose has a low Glycemic Index (GI) of 19 compared with 100 for glucose, yet it's much sweeter. Hence, they often recommend fructose as a sweetener for people with diabetes because it doesn't spike glucose and, subsequently, insulin level.

In the opposing corner, a growing number of scientists describe fructose as a toxin. Whom do we believe? Both sides are spilling truths, but only half the story. It's important to challenge what both are saying and get to the bottom by examining all the facts.

First, let's break down what the food industry says. Even though fructose has a low GI, it's true that too much fructose can damage the liver and increase triglycerides. It's not as benign as the food industry makes it out to be. That's why a growing number of scientists claim that fructose is a toxin. Still, that's a very strong statement to make!

The reality is, fructose is found naturally as a sweetener in fruits and other foods and is fine in normal doses. When you have too much fructose, that's when it becomes dangerous. Like anything in life, too much of something can render it hazardous. Take oxygen, for example. We need it to breathe, but did you know that too much oxygen can lead to brain cell death, convulsions, and even death?

Unfortunately, most people consume way too much fructose, thanks to something in many processed foods called high-fructose corn syrup. Before 1970, we used traditional sugar such as sugarcane or sugar beets to sweeten our foods. Recall that sugar or sucrose is a disaccharide that consists of a glucose binding to a fructose. Because half of sucrose is made of fructose (sweeter than glucose), it takes a lot more sugarcane and increases the cost to sweeten any foods. How could the food industry cut down cost and sweeten foods at the same time? The solution was high-fructose corn syrup (HFCS).

HFCS is derived from corn. Corn is milled to produce starch, which is further processed to break the starch into individual glucoses. Chemical enzymes are used to convert some of the glucose into fructose. Therefore, HFCS contains more fructose (55 percent) than glucose (42 percent). The remaining three percent is made up of large sugar molecules called saccharides.

Why do we use corn instead of other starches such as potatoes or rice? Why don't we have high-fructose rice syrup? The reason is very simple. It goes back to cost. Corn is easy to grow and cheap to produce. The US farm program subsidizes farmers to grow corn. After being genetically modified to resist drought and insects, corn is widely grown and harvested in the US A significant portion of corn is used only to make HFCS in the United States, making it the cheapest sweetener on the market. That's why you see so much HFCS added to almost all processed foods.

HFCS is transported as a liquid in large cylindrical trucks like gasoline. HFCS is widely used as a sweetener in sodas, juices, and sports drinks. It is also used to soften up baked goods and preserve the moisture for a long period of time since it doesn't crystallize or turn grainy when exposed to cold temperature. In addition, HFCS acts as a preservative to maintain freshness and extend shelf life to baked goods. That's why some cookies or cakes taste so fresh after being on the shelf for almost a year.

You can see why the food industry gravitates to HFCS to make everything we eat taste better by sweetening treats with fructose. From 1970 to 1990, the consumption of HFCS increased a whopping 1,000 percent. On average, Americans consume 60 pounds of the stuff every year. During the same period of time, the rate of obesity doubled from 15 percent in 1970 to 33 percent today. Is it mere coincidence?

Many researchers blame HFCS for the obesity epidemic. Before the development of the sugar industry, fructose was found only in a limited number of foods such as honey, dates, figs, and molasses. After the invention and commercial production of HFCS, the increased use of fructose to sweeten baked goods and common beverages, including soda, fruit juices, energy drinks, sports drinks, teas and coffees, has been documented to correlate directly with the obesity epidemic.

Consumption of sugary beverages has increased in the United States among both children and adults. According to data between 2005 to 2008 from the National Health and Nutrition Examination Survey, almost half of the US population drinks one sugary beverage on a given day, with at least one quarter drinking more than one 12-ounce can of soda. Teenagers and young adults consume more sugary drinks than any other group. Overweight and obese adolescents drink more than 300 calories per day, equaling an average of 15 percent of their total daily energy intake. According to a Harvard study, for each additional sugary soft drink consumed per day, participants gained an average of 1 pound over a four-year period. This is more weight gain than enjoying an extra serving of red meat per day. Sugary drinks have been linked to poor diet quality, weight gain, obesity, and type 2 diabetes in adults. The extra empty calories, along with the propensity for these sugary drinks to increase the insulin level, leads to fat storage and, ultimately, to weight gain.

A Princeton University research team led by Doctors Bartley G. Hoebel and Nicole M. Avena demonstrated that rats fed with HFCS gained significantly more weight than those with access to table sugar (sucrose), even when their overall caloric intake remained the same. The 2010 study, published in *Pharmacology, Biochemistry and Behavior*, also showed that long-term consumption of HFCS led to abnormal increases in abdominal fat and triglyceride level.

You may ask, "How can fructose increase triglyceride level?" It's because fructose isn't metabolized like glucose. Glucose is the universal source of energy for every living organism, so it's needed to power cells in vital organs such as our brain, heart, muscles, and kidneys. Glucose is absorbed into the cells via the transporting enzyme known as GLUT-4. But most cells don't have GLUT-5, the transporting enzyme for fructose. In fact, only liver cells have GLUT-5 to transport fructose. Hence, only the liver can use fructose.

Once transported inside the liver cells, fructose is quickly metabolized to become either glycogen or triglyceride, which is fat. The liver can only store a limited amount of glycogen. Once it reaches its maximum capacity, the rest of the fructose will be metabolized into fat. This fat will be transported and deposited all over the body.

Worse yet, HFCS makes you less full and hungrier. According to research conducted by the University of Pennsylvania, eating a high-fructose diet lowered the leptin level (not full) and elevated the ghrelin level (hungrier). Let's put it this way. Do you feel full drinking 32 ounces of soda or eating fries? They both contain about 500 calories, but you certainly would feel fuller with the fries. That's why sodas are considered *empty calories*. It's not that sodas are "empty" of calories. It just means calories from sodas count little as a nutrient to keep you full.

If soda isn't filling, why do we keep drinking it? To understand, you need to consider how the brain judges sugary drinks. Through many years of evolution, our brains have been wired to think that fluids contain only water. So when we look at a soda or begin to drink it, our brain sees the fluid as water rather than full of sugar. Sensing no sugar in water, our bodies are not prepared for the sudden rise in blood glucose that comes with sugary drinks. As a result, the pancreas is forced to release a massive amount of insulin quickly to deal with this sugar rush. High spikes in insulin will lead to dramatic drops in blood glucose, which can make us crave more sweets as our bodies try to compensate. As we feel hungry, we may grab something sweet or another soda, thus, repeating the cycle.

Sugar Is Addictive

We're hard-wired to love sweets. At the first bite of anything sweet, the monosaccharides glucose and fructose break down and stimulate the reward center in the brain, called the "nucleus accumbens," the same way cocaine and alcohol do. This causes a release of dopamine, the pleasure neurotransmitter. Over time, the body seeks more sugar in order to reinforce this feeling. Like alcohol and other drugs, sweets can be addictive as they may lead to withdrawal and tolerance. If you skip a soda, you might notice an intense craving for something sweet as your brain is withdrawing from sugar. But if you eat a lot of sweets, you'll develop tolerance over time. You might have to eat more sweets in order to get the same pleasure. We often see tolerance and withdrawal with alcohol, cocaine, morphine, and other stimulants.

Besides the fact that both are addictive, alcohol and fructose share a few similarities. In a study conducted by the University of California, San Francisco, researchers compared fructose with alcohol. The study, published in September 2010, points out that fructose metabolism is similar to alcohol. Alcohol is made from fermented glucose and fructose. Only the liver can metabolize fructose and alcohol. Therefore, the chronic consumption of fructose leads to the same diseases caused by chronic alcohol abuse.

Both alcohol and fructose abuse can cause high blood pressure. Alcohol drinkers were found to have a 30 percent increased risk of developing hypertension. Fructose causes salt retention and vasoconstriction that lead to hypertension. Excessive alcohol users have a higher risk of developing heart failure, while chronic fructose abusers are more likely to end up with a heart attack. Furthermore, both fructose abuse and alcohol abuse lead to elevated levels of triglycerides fat. Since both fructose and ethanol are high in calories, excessive consumption of both can lead to obesity.

While it's well known that excessive alcohol consumption causes many types of liver disease, multiple sources prove that fructose also causes fatty liver disease. Just like alcohol, fructose also causes pancreatitis. Chronic pancreatitis will eventually destroy beta cells, which are located in the pancreas to produce and store insulin. With the destruction of beta cells, there is an increased risk of developing type 2 diabetes, which is associated with both chronic alcoholism and chronic fructose consumption. With the increased risk of hypertension, high cholesterol, and type 2 diabetes, both fructose and alcohol cause metabolic syndrome.

As you're reading this, you must keep in mind that *too much* sugar, both glucose and fructose, can be detrimental to your health. We want to emphasize that it's the *amount*, rather than the sugar itself. To avoid potential problems with fructose and glucose, would artificial sweeteners be good alternatives?

THE TRUTH ABOUT ARTIFICIAL SWEETENERS

Chemists formulated artificial sweeteners as a way to circumvent problems associated with natural sugar. Artificial sweeteners are synthetic sugar substitutes that are many times sweeter than natural sugars. They're widely used in processed foods and in small packets placed in tea and coffee. According to the market research firm Mintel, a total of 3,920 products containing artificial sweeteners were launched in the United States between 2000 and 2005. In the US, there are five artificially derived sugar substitutes in the order of sweetness approved for use—aspartame, acesulfame potassium, saccharin, sucralose, and neotame.

Aspartame (NutraSweet®, Equal®) is the most popular sweetener in the US food industry. It's 180 times sweeter than regular sugar. Discovered accidentally in 1965, it's made from aspartic acid and phenylalanine, with a bit of methanol. More than two hundred million people worldwide consume aspartame. It's found in more than six thousand products, including dessert mixes, puddings, yogurt, chewing gums, and tabletop sweeteners. It's also found in sugar-free cough drops.

Acesulfame potassium (Sunett®, Sweet One®) is two hundred times sweeter than regular sugar. The ingredient is currently used in more than four thousand foods and beverages including candies, baked goods, frozen desserts, beverages, dessert mixes, and tabletop sweeteners in about ninety countries around the world. It's often combined with other sweeteners in well-known sodas (Diet Pepsi®, Coke Zero®, etc.) for a synergistic sweetening effect.

Saccharin (Sweet'N Low®, Sugar Twin®) is three hundred to five hundred times sweeter than regular sugar. Saccharin was discovered in 1879 by researchers at Johns Hopkins University. Saccharin is one of the most studied food ingredients, and is approved by the World Health Organization and thirty human studies. It is used in candy, baked goods, canned fruit, jams, chewing gum, dessert toppings, salad dressings, and tabletop sweeteners. It also works in cosmetic products and vitamins.

Sucralose (Splenda®) is six hundred times sweeter than regular sugar. It's made from real sugar. It was discovered in 1976 by chemically replacing three hydrogen-oxygen groups on the sucrose molecule with three chlorine atoms. Sucralose is found in over five thousand food products. Its safety profile consists of scientific studies conducted over twenty years. This sweetener is nontoxic, even at levels in animals that equal 40-plus pounds of sugar per day for life. It isn't metabolized by the body and has no known side effects.

Neotame (no brand names) is chemically similar to aspartame. The FDA approved neotame in 2002 after reviewing a hundred scientific safety studies. It's the sweetest of all—about seven thousand to thirteen thousand times sweeter than sugar. According to its website, neotame is the fastest-growing sweetener in the world. Neotame is a derivative of the dipeptide composed of the amino acids, aspartic acid, and phenylalanine.

Stevia (Truvia®, SweetLeaf®, NuNaturals, etc.) is a natural herbal extract from super sweet leaves that contain glycosides and many proteins and vitamins. The plant itself grows in Paraguay, where it has been used safely for the last fifteen hundred years. Stevia is about twenty-five to thirty times sweeter than sugar. Although it's been used worldwide for years, the FDA didn't "approve" its use until 2008. Actually, the FDA issued letters of "no objection," which means it won't object to companies using stevia in foods and beverages.

————

Artificial sweeteners do offer consumers some benefits. For one, they're much sweeter than regular sugar, but they don't behave like sugar in that they don't cause dental decay and cavities. Despite the sweetness, artificial sweeteners have virtually no calories and are used to sweeten diet sodas or sugar-free drinks. To give you a better perspective, each gram of regular sugar contains about four calories. So a regular 12-ounce can of soda contains about eight teaspoons of sugar, or about 130 calories. In addition, artificial sweeteners have been recommended as an alternative to sugar if you have diabetes because they don't raise the blood sugar level. In fact, many diet programs allow the use of sugar substitutes. High-protein bars often use sugar substitutes to make them taste sweet.

Although we've seen artificial sweeteners in the news for possible links to cancer, according to the National Cancer Institute and other health agencies, there's no scientific evidence that any of the five artificial sweeteners approved by the FDA cause any serious health problems, including cancer. They're considered safe in limited quantities, even for pregnant women. It's likely that a lot of the foods you eat contain some form of artificial sweetener.

The problem comes when you focus so much on the potential benefits of artificial sweeteners, you develop cognitive distortions to believe that you can have as many "sugar-free" juices or diet sodas as you want. A study looking at twenty-four thousand US adults found that overweight and obese adults who drank diet beverages consumed significantly more solid-food calories than those who drank sugary beverages. Not surprisingly, the study found that overweight and obese adults drank more diet beverages than healthy-weight adults. It's more than just calories that you have to worry about. Artificial sweeteners may worsen your sugar cravings.

Some research suggests that sugar substitutes don't satisfy your cravings like real sugar, potentially causing people to seek more and more diet drinks. In a 2008 study of women who drank water that was alternately sweetened with sugar and Splenda®, they could not tell the difference in taste, but their brains could. The functional MRIs showed that the brain reward system responded to both sugar and artificial sweeteners, but sugar lit up the brain's reward system more completely. The lead author of the study, Dr. Martin P. Paulus, a professor of psychiatry at the University of California, San Diego, suggested that diet sodas might be addicting because artificial sweeteners have positive reinforcing effects by triggering the brain's reward system. In other words, the brain knows it's not real sugar but it still wants the real thing, so it sends signals making you crave more sweets and carbohydrates. This might explain why at times you crave cookies, ice cream, and pasta. The "sugar-free" drinks might have zero calories, but your cravings for sweets and carbohydrates can be so strong that you'll end up eating more *total calories*. Yes, that means there's a higher risk for weight gain with even diet sodas or other zero-calorie drinks.

A recent study from the University of Texas Health Science Center at San Antonio found that diet soda drinkers have larger waistlines than nonusers. For nearly a decade, researchers compared the long-term change in waist circumference of diet soda users with nonusers, including those drinking regular sodas and those not drinking any soda. The result showed that diet soda drinkers have a 70 percent greater increase in belly bulge compared with nondiet drinkers. Those who drank two or more diet sodas per day were five times more likely to see an increase in their waist circumference than nondiet drinkers.

While the study showed a connection between diet soda consumption and an increased waistline, it didn't show that one caused the other. The true mechanism still remains unknown. Some studies suggest that when your taste buds sense sweetness, your body expects a calorie to accompany it. So when this doesn't happen, you overeat because you crave the energy rush your body is expecting.

In summary, regardless of the type of sweeteners used, you must view the HFCS or artificial sweeteners as occasional treats, rather than as a need at every meal. So much of your food and condiments are sweetened with either HFCS or artificial sweeteners, it's hard for you to avoid them altogether. In order to minimize the use of sweeteners, try your best to avoid any sweets. With Thinsulin, we teach you to group your foods into categories. One of the categories is sweets such as desserts, drinks, and snacks. We hope this background information will give you a better understanding of why you must avoid sweets during the Active Phase, and minimize their intake during the Passive Phase. After all, the truth about sweeteners isn't always so sweet.

PART III
THINSULIN PHASE ONE: THE ACTIVE PHASE

Sarah, a thirty-one-year-old mortgage broker, felt a serious lack of control over her weight. At her peak, she weighed 334 pounds on a 5'7" frame. This put her at a dangerously high BMI of 52.3. She knew she was at risk for other medical problems if she didn't lose weight. She contemplated weight-loss surgery but that was not her cup of tea. She could stay where she was, but that was too physically uncomfortable. She couldn't sleep, she felt sluggish, and she was in constant pain with a hurt back and an ache in her knees. She felt much older than her age due to her excess weight.

Sarah's brother told her about the Lorphen Medical Clinic in her city of Anaheim, California, in March 2015. Sarah decided to give it a try. The traditional approach to dieting had never worked for her, and she desperately needed a fresh opportunity to make changes in her life.

After all, Sarah had struggled with her weight for the past eleven years. Her weight had climbed steadily from stress, along with a psychological tipping point in the form of unhealthy relationships that kept driving her to overeat. The weight had been piling on since 2009.

"After every bad breakup, I would stop focusing on my health," Sarah shared. "I had a bad mindset. I knew I was gaining weight, but I just couldn't take action."

At a certain point, she felt she was "too far gone" to ever get down to the 150 pounds she had been at age twenty, so she collapsed into self-sabotage. Sarah's all-or-nothing thinking had made it impossible for her to take that giant step needed to change. Luckily, the principles of CBT (Cognitive Behavioral Therapy) central to the Thinsulin Program taught Sarah how to take small steps towards change.

For example, Sarah was quite intrigued with the role of insulin and weight loss until she learned that she needed to stay away from sweets. The thought of giving up sweets paralyzed her, provoking tremendous anxiety as she thought back to her upbringing.

Like most Americans, Sarah grew up eating traditional carbohydrates like rice, bread, and cheese. She now sees excess that at the time she viewed as normal. "I'd grab a piece of cheese, a piece of bread, and a hardboiled egg for breakfast and go," Sarah says. "I thought that's what all families ate for breakfast."

Dessert was also a familiar item in her household. "My dad has a very big sweet tooth, so we always had ice cream and cookies," says Sarah. That's not to say the refrigerator was empty of fruits and veggies, Sarah adds, but she didn't always make the best choices. "I clung to the sweeter things, and left behind the proteins and vegetables," she says.

Sweets were more than just a comfort food during times of stress. They became her best friend. When she was down, the ice cream or cake seemed to ease her sorrow. The more stress she had in her life, the more she turned to sweets to soothe her pain. So the thought of giving up sugars was understandably scary for her. Fear was written all over her face.

As she followed Thinsulin, Sarah realized that this program wasn't another diet. She needed to free herself from the monstrous cycle of punishment (giving up sweets), reward (cheating), and guilt (overeating) that had perpetuated her weight gain. The only solution was to change her thinking.

Cognitive Behavioral Therapy challenged her all-or-nothing thinking. She didn't have to give up sweets for the rest of her life. She only had to do it during the Active Phase for four months. When that still seemed too long to Sarah, she was asked to stay away from sweets to lower her insulin for only a week. One week was more realistic and doable.

This is such an important point. When it comes to weight loss, many people set goals that are out of reach. They expect that they can juice instead of eating solid foods, starve by eating only 500 calories per day, or go low-carb all the time. The mere thought of doing it is too daunting for them to even start. So they wait and push back that diet to another day.

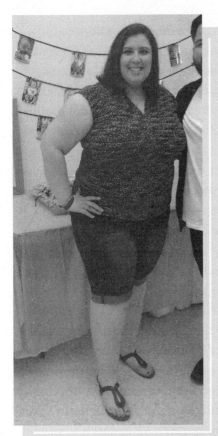

Sarah Before:
March 2015, 334 pounds

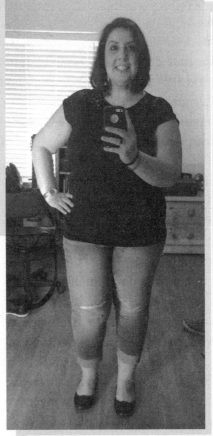

Sarah After:
July 2015, 271 pounds

By making goals more achievable, it seemed less scary for Sarah to take the next step. Certainly, she felt confident she could give up sweets for a week, especially when she knew that she was able to eat plenty of other foods that wouldn't spike her insulin level.

The first few days of the Active Phase were a bit uncomfortable as her body broke free from its addiction to carbs and sugars. But after one week, Sarah noticed her sugar cravings had diminished substantially. She was able to replace her bad habits with healthier ones through the principles of behavioral modification that are a signature of Thinsulin.

Sarah noticed that the Active Phase was kinder to her wallet than the fast food kings out there. Buying food for five satisfying meals a day that made fat melt off was infinitely more satisfying, too! She just had to make time to plan and prepare the meals. This gave her needed structure. "Before, I was eating out late," she says. "I learned that that was really bad for me. I don't do that now because I'm always full."

Sarah saw her weight drop right away. Every week, she saw more weight loss. What impressed her the most was how she began to view food differently. Her thinking changed. She didn't see food as her best friend or worst enemy. She was thinking in terms of insulin. That extra pressure of messing up and fearing the worst had vanished.

One month into the Active Phase, Sarah hit a minor snafu. She was having trouble drinking dairy-free black coffee due to the bitter taste. Still, she couldn't stop drinking coffee altogether because she needed her caffeine fix.

"I found caramel-flavored coffee, and I thought, Cool! And I kept drinking it," she said. "When I double-checked, I realized it was spiking my insulin. I tried to skate by, but now I've adjusted and refocused because I'm seeing huge results."

Sure enough, her weight loss stalled for three weeks. She didn't feel discouraged. She didn't want to give up for having had a small setback. She knew that this wasn't a short race to her destination, but a long haul in her journey. She enjoyed the process of thinking in terms of insulin.

"Before, I just wanted to get fast food because I didn't feel like cooking. Now, I've become a chef of sorts!" For the first time, she made cauliflower without frying it. She cooks spaghetti squash with shrimp. She cooks up veggies, puts a little salt and pepper on them, and throws them in the oven.

Thinsulin also gave her more freedom to choose. She didn't feel the constraints of eating only prepackaged foods. She's able to try out new restaurants and go to birthday parties and still lose weight.

Thinsulin has changed Sarah's life forever. She'll be faced with challenges along the way, but the reward at the end of this journey is simply too transformative to miss. She no longer dwells on her mistakes. Instead of blaming or shaming, she kept her eyes on the prize and moved forward. She didn't let those mistakes frustrate her and impede her progress. She realized that she has the skills and tools to succeed. Nothing can stop her now.

After four months on the Active Phase, Sarah has lost over 63 pounds. "It's so simple and easy. It's like magic. I'm not afraid of gaining back the weight because I understand now how it all works."

Chapter 6

SIMPLE FOOD CHOICES
THAT HELP YOU LOSE WEIGHT

Welcome to the Active Phase of the Thinsulin Program. In this phase, you'll spend the next four months lowering your insulin level so that your body will burn fat. Using principles of CBT (Cognitive Behavioral Therapy) and behavioral modifications, you'll learn to change your thinking and break bad habits. In the process, you can expect to lose at least 3 to 5 (and up to 10) pounds in the first week and about 5 percent of your total weight each month for a grand total of 20 percent at the end of four months. Some patients on Thinsulin have lost as much as 50 pounds in fifty days. Although it may sound difficult at first, you'll learn how to overcome challenges and discover a whole new you in your weight-loss journey.

Before we developed this program, back when we first began to educate our patients on how to eat the right foods, we would spend an hour talking in detail, basing our comments on the food pyramid. We even threw in notes from research articles to support our summation. We were quite proud of ourselves for being so complete. Even though the patient nodded throughout the talk and was even inquisitive throughout the discussion, we realized afterward that the information flew in one ear and out the other. Our thorough speech was utterly useless because it was total information overload for our patient. Had we highlighted a few basic guidelines for our patient to remember, we would have been more successful. We realized we had to find a better way to teach more effectively.

So we put ourselves in their shoes, which had been such a helpful tactic while working with the dancer Natalie, who was despondent at gaining weight from taking antipsychotic medications. This proved useful again. We realized the transformation from a concept to an action became undoable once our patients felt they had to give up all enjoyment in their life. For some, it might be a can of soda. For others, it could be potatoes or pasta. How long can you avoid going to dinner parties? Sometimes, you want to try a new restaurant. If you're counting calories, what and how much do you eat when you're at a restaurant? Do you just avoid social gatherings altogether if you've already used up all of a program's calories at lunchtime? You see, if a program is too strict, it's not sustainable forever. With Thinsulin, it's different. You don't have to give up all your enjoyment for the rest of your life.

We needed a program that would be realistic. Our goal has always been to offer you a program that realistically fits your schedule and needs. You can have all that if you learn to think in terms of insulin. When you're able to see foods in terms of insulin, it's up to you to choose what you want to do. Thinsulin empowers you to control your weight-loss journey.

Vidi is a twenty-seven-year-old married working mother who previously weighed 162 pounds on a petite 5′2″ frame. Like so many others who have found superior weight loss results on the Thinsulin Program, Vidi had tried many other methods to lose weight. Like her coworkers, she'd also tried fad diets, including drinking green juice for several months. "How long can I realistically drink this?" she asked herself. Sure enough, as soon as she stopped, she regained all her weight. She told us that Thinsulin has changed her life and her way of thinking. "Thinsulin is a more realistic way of losing weight," she told us. "It's not a diet." She described why the program works for her: "You don't have the mentality of restriction," she explains. "If you try to restrict me from something, I'm going to do it even more." Even though she has to avoid certain foods to prevent an insulin spike

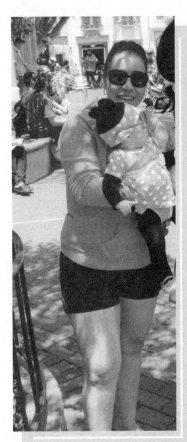

Vidi Before:
August 2014, 162 pounds

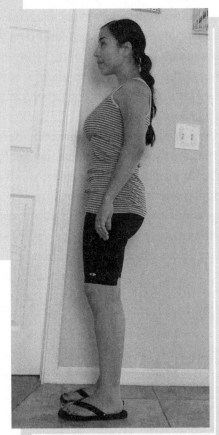

Vidi After:
August 2015, 134 pounds

during the Active Phase, she doesn't view it as a restriction. "I understand the effect of insulin on fat, so it's my choice to avoid those foods because I want to burn fat." Thinsulin helped Vidi keep her weight steady after one year at 134 pounds, a 17.3 percent weight loss.

So, how do you know which foods to eat and beverages to drink—and just as important, which to avoid? The Active Phase is all about living by one easy guideline: the Thinsulin Food Groups.

THE THINSULIN FOOD GROUPS

Although the glycemic index is a useful resource for determining whether or not an individual food will spike your insulin level, quite frankly, it's impossible to memorize thousands of individual foods and their glycemic index and glycemic load. So what we've done for you is simple. All you have to do is mentally break down what you're eating or drinking into five groups and understand how each group affects your insulin level.

As a kid, you probably learned about four food groups—grains, meats, dairy, and vegetables. With Thinsulin, we've modified the categories so that you can more quickly determine insulin response. Identify if what you want to eat falls under **sweets, fruits, grains, vegetables,** or **proteins**. Once you put the foods (or drinks) you want to consume into one of these five groups, it's much easier for you to know if the food will increase your insulin level.

SWEETS

Beverages

You may be surprised to learn how much sugar is found in typical drinks. A 20-ounce soda contains about seventeen packets of sugar; an Arizona Iced Tea contains roughly thirteen packets of sugar; and a Vitamin Water bottle contains approximately eight packets of sugar (as much as an 8-ounce can of soda. It's not just water with vitamins!).

As you consider beverages, ask yourself, "Will this drink spike my insulin level?" When it comes to beverages such as regular sodas, fruit juices, or sports drinks, the answer is a resounding "yes!" These drinks are very high in sugar. All sugary drinks will ultimately increase your insulin level, causing your body to store fat. You won't lose weight if you continue drinking sugary drinks.

What about using artificial sweeteners instead? You might think these are OK because they have zero calories and are sugar-free. From an insulin point of view, that's absolutely true, because artificial sweeteners *don't* spike the insulin level. But from a craving perspective, numerous scientific studies have shown that using artificial sweeteners actually makes you crave more carbohydrates and sugar. Even though artificial sweeteners are much sweeter than regular sugar, your brain knows they're not real sugar. Your brain doesn't like to be tricked. Your brain will signal to the area of the brain that controls craving, causing you to want more sugar and carbs. Therefore, at the end of the day, you'll end up eating more calories than you want. We don't recommend that you have any drinks that are sweet. That includes those sweetened with artificial sweeteners.

What can you drink, then, that won't spike your insulin level? Water is fine. What if you're tired of drinking plain water? You may consider adding lemon, lime, cucumber, or fresh mint to water. If you like the bubbly taste of sodas, you might want to try carbonated water, like seltzer or club soda. You just have to be careful because not all carbonated waters are the same. For example, a 12-ounce can of *tonic* water contains 32 grams of sugar and 124 calories.

How about unsweetened iced tea or hot tea? Sure! Tea has thousands of varieties to taste. The same goes for coffee. As long as you're not adding anything sweet, such as agave, honey, sugar, or artificial sweeteners, that would be fine.

Desserts

Any sweets such as desserts, snacks, or drinks will spike your insulin level. Therefore, we recommend you avoid them. Remember, you're not avoiding eating cakes, cookies, chocolate, and ice cream because of the empty calories or because they're junk food. We want you to go beyond that—be more specific and scientific. You're choosing not to eat sweets because they'll spike your insulin level. We want you to imagine the disappointment of that insulin spiking and your body storing fat *instead* of burning fat! It may sound tough as you're reading this to avoid desserts because they spike insulin during the Active Phase. Don't worry. It's not as hard as it seems. Thinsulin isn't a diet, so you're not left hungry. If you're able to eat twenty meatballs, will you feel full? Wouldn't it be easier for you then to walk away from that cheesecake? You have to avoid spiking your insulin only for four months during the Active Phase. It's not for the rest of your life.

Condiments and Sauces

Are you allowed to have any condiments and sauces? Be careful. High-fructose corn syrup is often used to sweeten them. If it tastes sweet, it probably has a lot of sugar. Use common sense. If you see honey BBQ sauce or sweet and sour sauce, that should give away the answer.

If you're going to use any sauces or condiments such as ketchup or mustard, dip them on the sides rather than drenching your dish with the sauce. You have much better control of how much you're going to dip than if you pour them all over your foods.

FRUITS

Instead of snacking on sweets, have a fruit as a morning snack. While all fruits contain sugars, some are more likely than others to cause your insulin level to spike. Remember, Glycemic Index measures the effect that foods have on blood glucose. Avoid eating high-Glycemic Index (GI) fruits such as watermelon, pineapples, bananas, and cantaloupes. You may have low-GI fruits, but limit your portion size. Eating more than one portion size per serving will increase your insulin level.

The good news is that there are many low-GI fruits you can have. But to make it simple and easy to remember, you may have a portion of an **apple**, **orange**, **grapes,** or **berries** (such as cherries, raspberries, blueberries, blackberries, or strawberries). A portion is about the size of your fist. When you take into account all the different types of these fruits, there are a lot more choices than you think!

The fruits you eat must be fresh and in the form of whole foods, as dried, processed, or canned fruits contain a lot more sugar. That means dried fruits such as raisins, and processed foods like strawberry yogurts, are out. You may get a plain yogurt and add fresh strawberries to it, but you can't buy the one with strawberries already in it. You also need to stick to eating these fruits only in the morning as a snack because they aren't as filling as nuts. If a fruit is eaten as an afternoon snack, it might not hold you until dinner compared with a handful of raw nuts.

Again, it's important to think in terms of insulin. If you think in terms of what seems healthy, you might be missing an important point. For example, if you play sports, you've probably been told to eat bananas in order to prevent muscle cramps. Unfortunately, a banana is a high-GI fruit that will spike your insulin level. If you eat bananas, your body won't be able to burn fat.

It can be overwhelming to learn all the fruits that can spike your insulin level. How could anyone memorize such a long list? You don't have to. Once you identify what you're eating as a fruit, you just have to repeat to yourself, "*Apple, orange, grapes, or berries.*" As long as you eat one portion of these four fruits as a morning snack a day, you won't spike your insulin level.

Some of you may be wondering about other low-GI fruits like avocados. You might reason that avocados don't spike your insulin level, so they should be allowed. Learning from our lessons, the key to success is to keep the program simple. If you only have to remember four fruits that you can eat, you can focus more on learning the technique of grouping the foods, rather than trying to figure out the GI of each fruit you want to eat. Just keep it simple. Don't deviate beyond the four fruits—remember your mantra: apple, orange, grapes, or berries.

In addition, apples are a great source of fiber, containing both soluble and insoluble fiber, which keep you feeling full. Perhaps that's what the old saying, "An apple a day keeps the doctor away" is *really* talking about.

GRAINS

Grains should be avoided during the Active Phase if you want to burn fat by lowering your insulin level. *Any* grains will cause your insulin to spike.

Grains such as wheat, barley, oats, and rice are complex carbohydrates composed of long complex chains of simple sugars that break apart upon digestion to provide us with energy. Grains are used to make flour, breads, buns, pasta, pizza, cereal, crackers, biscuits, cookies, and cakes. Grains are packed with high calories and tend to raise blood sugar as well.

Anything made out of grains will cause an increase in your insulin level. This includes bread, cereal, oatmeal, bagels, crackers, noodles, pasta, pizza, tortillas, and rice. Even though brown rice or wheat bread is thought to be nutritional, they're somewhat tricky foods because they'll still cause your insulin level to spike, and will thus prevent weight loss.

Many studies have shown that eating low-GI foods, such as wheat bread and brown rice, offers numerous health benefits in patients with diabetes. However, the Glycemic Load of both multigrain breads and brown rice is high, thus they will increase your insulin level. In order to lower your insulin level, you must avoid eating breads (wheat or white), tortillas, pasta, pizza, cereals, crackers, biscuits, cookies, cakes, noodles, and rice (brown or white).

When we share this advice, we often get a lot of pushback. Nutritionists have taught you that multigrain breads and brown rice are healthy and should be part of your diet. The question isn't whether or not multigrain breads or brown rice are healthy for you. The question is, do healthy grains spike your insulin level? The answer is a resounding yes!

Over two hundred million Americans eat products made of wheat daily. Dr. William Davis, author of *Wheat Belly*, recommends dropping wheat from your diet entirely in order to lose weight and gain health. Even wheat will spike your insulin level. So if you eliminate wheat from your diet, your insulin level will drop.

If you're not convinced, here's another example. What is beer made of? If you guessed barley, wheat, or grains, you're absolutely correct. Barley, wheat, or grains increase insulin, thus causing the body to stop burning existing fat and instead store excess calories into fat. Where does this fat go? Everywhere, but especially your belly. That's why you often see "beer bellies," but you rarely see "wine bellies." What are wines made from? You guessed it, grapes! Remember, grapes are low-GI fruits. Therefore, you're unlikely to develop a "wine belly" as long as you have no more than a glass per day. You might blame calories for a beer gut, but it's really the grains that beer is made from that spike insulin level, leading the body to store fat in the belly.

Again, it's important to think beyond what you've heard is "healthy" when choosing your foods. Take a look at veggie burgers: so many of our patients choose veggie burgers over beef patties for "health" reasons. What they don't realize is how much *wheat* is added to veggie burgers! Eating veggie burgers will spike your insulin level, so that won't help your waistline.

When you consider that an average American consumes almost 2,000 pounds of grains yearly, you can see why we have an obesity epidemic.

Some people prefer quinoa as their healthy choice. Even though quinoa is an insoluble fiber, it has a GI of 53 and GL of 13 so it still can spike the insulin level. We recommend avoiding quinoa during the Active Phase.

VEGETABLES

Looking at the salad bar? You can pretty much eat any vegetables you want, except for starchy vegetables such as potatoes, corn, carrots, and beets. A simple cue to remember which veggies to eat is this singsong couplet:

"Potatoes, corn, carrots, and beets, these are the veggies I cannot eat."

On the other hand, spinach, kale, lettuce, asparagus, celery, bok choy, cauliflower, cucumber, mushrooms, tomatoes, and peppers, and leafy green vegetables in general are all great choices on the Thinsulin Program.

A plant's leaves are green because they contain chlorophyll, so that they can perform photosynthesis to produce glucose. Leaves and other flowering parts of the plants typically don't store starch, so their GI is low.

A plant's sugar is stored in the form of starch in the roots (carrots, parsnips, and radishes), tubers (potatoes and yams), or kernels (corn) of the plants. It's best to avoid these during the Active Phase.

Potatoes may surprise you as a "problem food" as they have been an important part of the human diet for thousands of years. They do have some good qualities; they are still certified as a "heart healthy" food by the American Heart Association, and are a good source of vitamin C, several B vitamins, and minerals, including potassium, magnesium, phosphorus, and iron. But many people don't realize the impact of potatoes on insulin. The problem is how much most people tend to consume. For that reason, it's best to avoid them altogether on the Active Phase.

It's commonplace to serve potatoes in several different forms with our meals, including hash browns for breakfast, French fries for lunch, potato chips for a quick snack, and mashed or baked potatoes for dinner. According to data from the US Department of Agriculture, a typical American consumes 130 pounds of potatoes each year. That's a lot of potatoes!

A study from Harvard Medical School published in the *New England Journal of Medicine* examined more than a hundred twenty thousand American men and women over a twelve- to twenty-year period and found that people who ate an extra serving of French fries or potato chips every day gained an average of 3.35 pounds and

1.69 pounds respectively over a four-year period. Over a twenty-year period, the average weight gain reached 16.8 pounds. This might explain weight gain as we get older. The study further showed that the daily consumption of an extra serving of potatoes caused more weight gain than having an additional 12-ounce serving of a sugar-sweetened drink or eating an extra portion of unprocessed red meat.

Potatoes are very high in carbohydrates and will cause a rapid rise in blood sugar levels. In addition, potatoes pack a lot of calories. A large serving of French fries contains between 500 to 600 calories, while a large baked potato (without any condiments) contains about 275 calories. The bottom line is to stay away from potatoes, even sweet potatoes such as yams, while you're lowering your insulin level.

Corn has been another staple of the American diet for many years. It's associated with the Midwest and could be considered the vegetable equivalent of apple pie. Yet look closer and you'll see that corn is high in carbohydrates and will elevate the insulin level, so it should be avoided when you're trying to lose weight.

Many people believe beets are healthy. They often throw beets into their juicer along with other vegetables to make healthy juices. They don't realize that beets are very high in sugar, and thus, will increase insulin. In fact, most table sugars are made from either sugarcanes or beets.

There's a debate on whether carrots are considered low- or high-GI vegetables and thus, whether or not you should avoid them. Rather than memorizing each individual vegetable and its effect on insulin, we want to make it simple for you to remember. Plants don't store starch in leaves or flowering parts, but they do store starch in roots, tubers, and kernels. What does starch do to insulin? It will spike your insulin level, causing your body to store fat. On the other hand, green, leafy vegetables are made from cellulose or fiber, so they won't spike your insulin level. Plus, the high fiber helps you feel full and reduces constipation.

In general, fresh vegetables are always better than canned or processed vegetables because they don't have any additional ingredients (such as high-fructose corn syrup that so often sneaks into canned items). Raw, uncooked vegetables tend to have more nutrients than cooked vegetables, so try to have at least one meal per day with uncooked vegetables. And by repeating the singsong rhyme, you're reminding yourself to simply avoid vegetables that store starch in the roots, tubers, or kernels. You need to eat green, leafy vegetables, but you can have other vegetables as well.

PROTEINS

Proteins are insulin-safe foods because they have few, if any, carbohydrates. Proteins include meat, seafood, egg whites, dairy products, beans, and nuts.

Beef, Fowl, Seafood, Tofu, and Egg Whites. Dieters often attempt to eat less meat because they believe they'll lose weight faster. Unfortunately, doing this backfires because they often become so ravenously hungry that they resort to quick snacking on chips, cookies, or other high-carb snacks in order to quell their hunger. Truthfully, if you want to lose weight, you have to increase your protein intake. It has to do with balance. Add more beef, fowl, seafood, tofu, or egg whites to your diet. Meat such as beef or pork; poultry such as turkey, duck, and chicken; fish such as salmon or halibut; shellfish such as lobster or shrimp; and non-meats such as egg whites and tofu are high in protein and very low in carbs.

Foods high in protein will keep you full without increasing your insulin level. By avoiding carbs and eating a high-protein diet, you'll lower your insulin level and allow your body to burn fat.

Use common sense when you're eating more meat as a source of protein. You don't want to lower your insulin level at the expense of worsening your cholesterol levels. Choose lean meats and minimize eating skins if possible. You may eat red meat such as pork and beef, but you certainly don't want to eat them every day. This will only worsen your lipids and cholesterol levels, putting you at risk for a heart attack or stroke. Try to eat more chicken, turkey, and fish. To mix up the protein, you may also eat shellfish such as lobster and shrimp or other seafood. As for eggs, try to eat egg white rather than the whole egg that contains the yolk. Egg white is fat-free and high in protein, containing about 16 calories. Egg yolk is high in fat and nutrients, containing about 72 calories. If you do the math, you'll see a four-egg-white omelet has less calories than one whole egg omelet. You'll certainly feel fuller eating the egg white omelet. Since you can get plenty of nutrients with green, leafy vegetables, you want to eat mainly protein to help keep you full.

Dairy Products. Dairy products are typically high in protein and low in carbohydrates. Opt for cheese and Greek yogurt over milk or regular yogurt, and limit dairy only to breakfast. Skim or full-fat milk can spike insulin level almost as much as a slice of white bread. Although butter and cream don't spike insulin levels, they are both high in saturated fat, so use in moderation.

Compared with milk, most cheeses contain few carbohydrates. A cup of 1 or 2 percent fat milk contains about 13 grams of carbohydrates due to the natural sugar, lactose. While cheese is made from milk, the lactose is generally broken down by bacteria during the fermentation process, and cheese is left without any sugar.

Yogurt is made from fermented milk but is often flavored with sugar, which adds between 15 to 20 grams of carbohydrates per one-cup serving. Greek yogurt is also made from fermented milk, but it tends to be more concentrated with a thicker consistency. Compared with American yogurt, Greek yogurt contains more protein, less sugar, and fewer carbs per serving. This is why plain, unflavored Greek yogurt is preferred. Greek yogurt with added flavorings contain sugar that can spike your insulin level.

Even though dairy products are high in protein and low in carbs, we often notice that patients who add cheese to everything find it more difficult to lose weight. To limit the total caloric intake from dairy products, we have found it best that all dairy products be consumed *only* at breakfast and at no other meals. This is a very simple rule to remember. Who wants to eat creamy sauce or ranch dressing for breakfast? That's exactly why we keep it at breakfast only.

Beans, Tofu, and Nuts. Vegetarians will still need to have lots of protein for lunch and dinner, and beans and tofu are good sources. If you're not a vegetarian, try to eat more meat, egg whites, or seafood because they tend to keep you fuller for a longer time than beans. Beans and nuts are high in protein, but they're also packed with carbohydrates, although they have a low GI.

According to an article in the September 2008 *Journal of Nutrition*, nuts are very filling and don't lead to weight gain when you limit your portion to a fistful. Any more than that may lead to weight gain because they contain carbohydrates and high amounts of fat and calories.

You should always choose raw nuts. If you want roasted nuts, choose the dry roasted nuts over those roasted in oil. The ideal nuts contain less than two grams of saturated fat, or 10 percent of the daily value, per serving. Also, eat only one portion of nuts as an afternoon snack between lunch and dinner and no other time. Nuts will keep you full until dinner compared with fruits. Let's review which nuts you can have.

An ounce of pecans contains 3.8 grams of carbohydrates, but 2.7 grams of the carbohydrates are fiber. Therefore, your body is unable to digest fiber, so much of the fiber will pass through your digestive tract. The net gain for carbohydrates is 1.9 grams, making pecans suitable as an afternoon snack. Unfortunately, pecans are relatively high in calories—approximately 200 calories per 1-ounce serving.

An ounce of walnuts contains about 185 calories and 3.9 grams of carbohydrates, including 1.9 grams of fiber. The net gain for carbohydrates is 2 grams. Walnuts are also a good source of phosphorus (important for forming ATP or energy) and magnesium (needed for producing energy).

Hazelnuts are high in magnesium and vitamin E, which is an antioxidant that can limit cell damage from free radicals. Each ounce of hazelnuts contain 5 grams of carbohydrates, including 2.7 grams of fiber. The net gain of carbohydrates is 2.3 grams, so it's a little higher than the recommended intake. An ounce of hazelnuts contains about 183 calories.

Almonds have a GI of zero, but they have 6 grams of carbohydrates, including 3.1 grams of fiber. The net gain of carbohydrates is 2.9 grams. Almonds contain roughly 170 calories per 1-ounce serving. Wonderfully rich in nutrients, almonds contain magnesium, phosphorus, and vitamin E.

Peanuts have a low GI as well as GL, so they're good to eat as snacks. While technically a legume instead of a nut, an ounce of peanuts contain a total of 6.1 grams of carbohydrates, including 2.3 grams of fiber. The net gain for carbohydrates is 3.8 grams. Peanuts contain about 166 calories per 1-ounce serving. They're also a good source for magnesium, phosphorus, and vitamin E.

Now that you know the five food groups and how they affect insulin levels, it's important to assess whatever you're eating or drinking: sweets, grains, vegetables, fruits, and proteins.

As you look at the diagram, you can see that the three circles resemble a traffic light. *Red* means you have to STOP. Don't eat *any* sweets, grains, or starchy vegetables because even a little bit of these foods can spike your insulin level.

Yellow indicates that you need to be CAUTIOUS. These are foods that are safe in moderation. Apples, oranges, grapes, and berries each have a low GI, so they're unlikely to spike one's insulin level as long as you have only one portion per day. Let's say

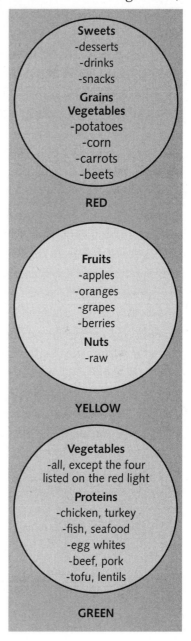

Sweets
-desserts
-drinks
-snacks
Grains
Vegetables
-potatoes
-corn
-carrots
-beets

RED

Fruits
-apples
-oranges
-grapes
-berries
Nuts
-raw

YELLOW

Vegetables
-all, except the four listed on the red light
Proteins
-chicken, turkey
-fish, seafood
-egg whites
-beef, pork
-tofu, lentils

GREEN

you try to eat "healthy" by having two oranges a day instead of eating junk food, not realizing that the two oranges have enough sugar to spike your insulin level. This is why you can have only one fresh fruit a day and only one portion of raw nuts per day for similar reasons. Nuts have some carbohydrates, but if you eat only one handful per day, this won't spike your insulin level.

Green means GO! These foods don't spike your insulin level, so you can have as much protein such as meat, seafood, and egg whites as you want. Make sure to eat plenty of green, leafy vegetables, too, because they don't spike insulin level due to the high fiber content.

––––––––

In summary, the Thinsulin food groups teach you to look beyond nutritional claims you may have heard from product companies and media sources about the relative health of foods, and instead, just think about foods in terms of how they affect insulin. Whenever you're faced with foods to choose from, simply categorize them into five groups—sweets, fruits, grains, vegetables, or proteins. Sweets and grains are pretty straightforward because they'll spike your insulin level. Avoid eating those. Once you've identified foods as either vegetables or fruits, just remember that you can eat all vegetables except for four—potatoes, corn, carrots, and beets. On the other hand, you can eat only four fruits—apple, orange, grapes, or berries—and no others. You can have all protein, such as meat, seafood, chicken, or egg whites, because they barely spike insulin. It's that simple!

Chapter 7

EAT MORE AND
STILL LOSE WEIGHT

N ow that you know which groups of foods to eat and which to avoid, what does this look like on a daily basis?

You've been on diets that leave you hungry, perhaps using prepackaged meals or replacement shakes to hold you over between breakfast, lunch, and dinner. Sometimes you might skip a meal, thinking that eating less will help you lose weight. But the truth is that it won't.

A critical rule in the Active Phase is to *avoid starving yourself.* In fact, you need to eat five meals a day. If you're hungry, you'll have to eat more food, rather than less, but you'll eat only foods that don't increase your insulin level. You will no longer need to count calories. All you'll do is eat enough protein and green, leafy vegetables to ensure that you're full.

You won't find set menus in this book for several reasons. First, what we select might not be what you want or even like to eat. Everyone has different tastes, and one of the highlights of the Thinsulin Program is that it works for everyone, regardless of one's food preferences.

Second, we know it's impossible for you to cook all of your meals. You'll have parties and dinners at your favorite restaurants, and you might have to eat out at work for lunch and/or dinner. That makes preset menus impractical at best and useless at worst.

Most important, though, is for you to learn the concepts of the program and apply them to your daily life. Doing that will ensure that your weight will stay off forever!

So instead of giving you specific menus, we'll provide an overall meal plan guide to help you lower your insulin level. That way you can mix and match your favorite foods with whatever you're in the mood to eat. Here are the general guidelines that will help you to do that.

Note: One portion is the size of your fist.

Breakfast

Protein—such as egg whites, sausage, chicken, etc.—or one portion of dairy product, such as plain, nonfat Greek yogurt or cottage cheese

Morning Snack

1 apple or orange or 1 portion of grapes or berries

Lunch

At least 1 portion each of protein and vegetables

Afternoon Snack

1 portion of nuts

Dinner

At least 1 portion each of protein and vegetables

BREAKFAST

Some people skip breakfast because they don't have time to eat in the morning. Others skip it because they're trying to lose weight. Lately, you may have heard some nutritionists advising skipping breakfast as a weight-loss tool, and some of us have tried it. Ultimately, it doesn't work. In fact, the opposite is true.

If you want to lose weight, you must eat breakfast every morning. Eating breakfast reduces your hunger later in the day, which helps you avoid overeating. Studies have shown that when you skip breakfast, you're more tempted to reach for a quick fix, such as a free doughnut in the break room or candy from a vending machine. Having fewer but larger meals isn't good because it fluctuates your insulin level. Eating smaller portions more frequently throughout the day helps stabilize your insulin level, which, as we've seen, helps your body burn fat more easily.

But worst of all, your body goes into starvation mode when you go hours without eating, especially when you skip breakfast, and it will store whatever you eat after that as fat.

You can eat any food for breakfast as long as it doesn't increase your insulin level. This may contradict what you learned as a kid. How can eggs be healthier than oatmeal or a banana? Remember: the goal is to lower your insulin level. Bananas and oatmeal are high in sugar and carbs, so they will increase your insulin. Proteins, such as eggs, won't. You can have them soft-boiled, hard-boiled, scrambled, or as omelets filled with vegetables. Remember to only eat egg whites and *not* the yolk.

Besides eggs, you can eat a plain, nonfat Greek yogurt or cottage cheese for breakfast. Dairy products are generally high in protein and low in carbs. You'll end up eating fewer calories for the day by avoiding dairy products like extra cheese, ranch dressings, or creamy sauce at lunch or dinner. Avoid drinking milk because it contains lactose, which your body recognizes and processes as sugar. A great alternative to cow's milk is unsweetened almond milk, which has no sugar in it and a lot more calcium.

If you're tired of eating eggs, Greek yogurt, and cottage cheese, have another protein—such as ham, sausage, or turkey—for breakfast, as long as it's not prepared with a sugary glaze that will raise your insulin level.

Our bodies react to the same foods differently depending on the time of day. Researchers have reported that the same food eaten for lunch causes less glucose response than when eaten for breakfast. This is why it's important to eat proteins for breakfast.

MORNING SNACK

Between breakfast and lunch, your first snack should always be a low-GI fruit, such as an apple, orange, grapes, or berries. These fruits do contain natural sugar, but eating one portion of any of them—the size of your fist—won't cause your insulin to spike. Two or more per day, however, and your insulin will rise, meaning you won't lose weight.

Maria was diagnosed recently with type 2 diabetes and came to our office hoping that losing weight might help her diabetic condition improve. She started the Thinsulin Program and did very well the first month, losing 20 pounds. But after her second month, she lost only 1 pound. She said that she was eating healthfully and was following the plan. But her food log told a different story: she was eating three oranges as her morning snack and two more in the evening.

Maria thought that, because oranges are healthy, having more of something healthy would be better than a bag of chips. She was right as far as the chips go, but eating more than one orange increased her insulin level and prevented her from losing more weight.

Maria's story isn't uncommon. When you understand and apply insulin level to what you eat, you'll have much greater success.

AFTERNOON SNACK

Between lunch and dinner, have a handful of raw nuts. Nuts are very filling and will prevent you from overeating before dinner. How many times have you felt so hungry after work that you snack on anything in sight while preparing dinner? When dinner's ready, though, you're so full from snacking that you skip most of it. But then, by the time you go to bed, your stomach is growling because you haven't eaten enough. Instead of eating a proper meal, you down a bowl of cereal and milk as a late-night snack. Cereal doesn't seem like a full meal and wheat cereals seem relatively healthy. But the carbs in the cereal plus the sugar in the milk will cause a huge spike in your insulin level.

Nuts are the answer. One handful as an afternoon snack has enough protein and fat to keep you full, but not enough carbs to increase your insulin level. You'll feel full until dinner is ready. Almonds and pistachios, which both have a GI of zero, are preferred. If you're allergic to tree nuts, try sunflower seeds. But keep fruit as your morning snack and nuts as your afternoon snack. Don't switch the order. Fruit isn't filling enough to hold you over until dinner.

LUNCH AND DINNER

For both lunch and dinner, you need to eat vegetables and proteins, such as meat, seafood, or tofu. You can eat as many green, leafy vegetables as you want as long as you avoid potatoes, corn, carrots, and beets.

As you can imagine, as you eat fiber that can't be digested, the fiber expands in your stomach to give you the sensation of fullness. Therefore, we recommend that you eat your green, leafy vegetables before you eat your proteins.

As a rule of thumb, the greener the vegetable, the more nutritious it is. Green leafy vegetables, such as asparagus, celery, cucumbers, lettuce, or spinach, don't have much sugar and are excellent sources of fiber. You can also prepare them many different ways. You don't always have to eat a salad to get your greens. Try them grilled, steamed, or sautéed with oil. Just don't use corn oil.

Dieters often believe that eating less or no meat will make them lose weight. But, again, the opposite occurs because they feel so hungry that they wind up snacking on potato chips, cookies, or granola bars. It's very important to eat *at least* one portion of meat, fowl, seafood, or tofu for lunch and for dinner. When you do, you'll feel fuller longer. You can eat more than one portion if you're not full after a meal. Also, pork, beef, chicken, or turkey will keep you feeling fuller longer than seafood or tofu. For those last two, you may want to plan to eat more than one portion in order to stay full.

As with vegetables, you can prepare the meat, seafood, or tofu in different ways. You don't always have to eat them steamed or broiled. You can use olive oil to sauté your meat. You can even eat deep-fried meat or seafood, but make sure neither is breaded. Eating fried foods once every few months is OK, but for obvious health reasons you should avoid eating them regularly due to the high saturated fats. Eating too much saturated fat increases the risks for heart attacks and strokes.

White meat, such as chicken, turkey, and fish, are healthier choices, but don't limit yourself to white meat alone. Mix it up! Don't eat the same boring food every day. Rub your protein with different spices, but be careful when marinating your meat with steak sauce or barbecue sauce because they have a lot of sugar, which will spike your insulin level. You can even use condiments, such as ketchup, mustard, or relish. You might be wondering, *Wait, can I really eat these condiments? The labels show that they're high in sugar and carbs.* You're absolutely correct, but remember: you aren't avoiding *all* carbs. If that were the case, you'd be avoiding fruits (high in sugar) and beans (high in carbs). The goal here is to lower your insulin level. Those sauces and condiments have sugar, like low-GI fruits, but the sugar content in them isn't high enough to increase your insulin level— as long as you don't use too much. How much is too much? As always, use common sense. Don't use any sauces that contain honey or added sugars, including honey barbeque and sweet-and-sour sauce. The "sweet" and "honey" in the names are the red flags that they will increase your insulin level.

Let's review: by eating three core meals—breakfast, lunch, and dinner filled with proteins and vegetables—with a low-GI fruit as a morning snack and a handful of nuts as an afternoon snack, you'll be less likely to cheat while you're lowering your insulin level so that your body will burn fat and lose weight.

Now, let's take what you've learned and apply it to real-life situations. Remember, don't cheat or starve yourself when you're lowering your insulin level. It's important to break down problem foods into the five groups—sweets, fruits, grains, vegetables, and proteins—and go from there.

EXAMPLE #1

You're at a birthday lunch where they're serving fish tacos. On the table sit chips, salsa, guacamole, and mango salsa for the fish tacos. What can you eat? Take a moment to think about it first before you continue reading.

Let's break down the fish taco first. The fish isn't breaded and is topped with purple cabbage, cilantro, and tomatoes. The taco shell is made of corn meal, so you can't eat that. The cabbage, cilantro, and tomatoes are vegetables—and not the four vegetables that you can't eat—so you can eat everything except the taco shell. (Botanists consider tomato as a fruit, but its genome turns out to be a vegetable. For simplicity, let's consider a tomato a vegetable because we often eat it like a vegetable.) You have to eat at least your fist-size portion of meat for lunch, so you'll need to eat at least two fish tacos, without the shells, to be full.

What about the salsas and guacamole? Again, break down what's in them. The salsa for the chips consists of tomatoes, onions, peppers, and cilantros—all good vegetables—so that's OK to eat. But mango isn't one of the four fruits that you can eat (apple, orange, grapes, or berries). The guacamole is made from avocados, tomatoes, cilantro, and lime. You know that you can eat the tomatoes and cilantro, so that's fine, but what about the avocado? Avocado is high in protein and fat, and low in carbs but it's technically a fruit. Similar to mango, you can't eat guacamole because avocado isn't one of the four fruits that you can eat. Just keep it simple!

As long as you think in terms of insulin, you don't have to limit yourself to the same foods every day. In fact, we don't want you to do that. We have many patients who successfully lose weight during a honeymoon cruise or extended vacation. They can eat at whichever restaurants they want by choosing foods that don't increase their insulin level.

EXAMPLE #2

Your best friend wants to celebrate in Las Vegas. The group decides on a buffet dinner. You paid good money for the buffet, so you want to get your money's worth. What can you eat?

Remember to break down the foods into the five groups: sweets, fruits, grains, vegetables, and proteins. You look around and see a lot of proteins—turkey, ham, shrimp, crab legs, steak, sausage, and beef. You know that these proteins won't increase your insulin level, so you can have at least fist-size portions of any of those. But you'll want to avoid the sweets, so no desserts or fruit (since you're at dinner). Also, stay away from the pasta and bread, which will spike your insulin level. This includes egg rolls because of the rice flour wrappers.

For the most part, you can eat as many vegetables as you want. Just remember the four veggies to avoid: potatoes, corn, carrots, and beets. So, you can have the green salad, asparagus, and tomatoes, for example, but stay away from the mashed potatoes.

EXAMPLE #3

It's a cold and rainy Sunday afternoon at home. You want something to warm you up, and vegetable soup would really hit the spot. Can you eat it?

Again, let's break it down. It has carrots, potatoes, onions, celery, corn, and parsley leaves. You know that you can't have potatoes, corn, or carrots, so you eat around them. That's OK, right?

This is the trouble with soup. When carrots and potatoes are cooked in a soup, the sugar in them releases into the broth. So even if you avoid eating the carrots, corn, and potatoes, your insulin level will still rise due to the increased sugar content in the broth.

Unfortunately, you can't have that vegetable soup, but the good news is that you can have chicken soup with green vegetables and without the noodles instead. This is a good example of thinking in terms of insulin.

As you can see, it's very simple to do the Thinsulin Program. Over time, you can train yourself to see all food in terms of insulin. You can quickly scan foods at any time, any place, and in any language and categorize them with the four problem groups to figure out immediately what you can eat that won't spike your insulin level. In this way, you control your weight for the long haul, and you'll watch in wonder as it stops controlling you.

Chapter 8

THE IMPORTANCE OF EXERCISE

What role does exercise play in the Thinsulin Program? Exercise is an integral part of any weight-loss program. You probably already know this, but motivating yourself to exercise is the difficult part. If you're going to the gym regularly, you expect to lose weight, but oftentimes you see minimal weight loss. You might think, "Ah, well, muscle weighs more than fat." That seems plausible, but the reality is, you're not building up that much muscle to keep your scale unchanged.

So why aren't you losing weight if you're exercising? Isn't exercise supposed to keep your heart healthy and burn off calories? Absolutely! The mistake you might make is thinking of exercise as part of the calories equation, rather than as part of the insulin equation. If you go on a four-mile jog and then eat exactly the same way you used to—snacking on cookies, eating desserts, and drinking sports drinks—can you expect to lose any weight? Not likely. In fact, if you believe you can have a slice of pecan pie because you ran on the treadmill earlier, ask yourself how long you have to run to burn off the calories of one slice of pecan pie? Yes, you have to jog roughly an hour to burn off 500 calories. If you're, say, enjoying a slice of cheesecake from the Cheesecake Factory, be prepared to jog for three hours!

You might have heard the saying, "Six-packs aren't made at the gym. They're made in the kitchen." What you eat will help burn fat more than the exercise you do at the gym. You might lift weights or do core exercises. You might get bigger and stronger, but not necessarily more toned. Muscles are hidden beneath layers of fat. The best way to naturally burn fat is to lower your insulin level. Imagine the results if you combine Thinsulin with exercise? You'll have the most success if you eat in a way to lower your insulin level and exercise consistently—roughly three times a week. If you can afford a personal trainer, he or she will help keep you on track and show you how to exercise properly and eat right.

EXERCISE IN THE ACTIVE PHASE

Let's discuss how Thinsulin relates to exercise. Likely, each of you has a different level of physical activity. Some of you might be physically inactive due to various factors: your joints might hurt too much for you to exercise due to your weight. At the other extreme, some of you might be very physically active. You might be jogging, biking, or taking kickboxing classes. The rest of you are somewhere in-between.

If you're exercising, that's awesome! Don't even think about stopping. Continue to exercise throughout the Active Phase. If you do aerobic exercise or cardio workouts, you might wonder if you're eating enough carbs with Thinsulin. It depends on how much exercise you're doing. If you're running a marathon, then, yes, you'll need to load up on grains. But, most likely, your exercise intensity is not to that level. Remember, you're not starving while on the Thinsulin Program. You're still eating dairy in the morning, vegetables, fruit, and then nuts as your snacks. You're eating carbohydrates that will break down to glucose and power your body. Plus, you're still eating proteins to help you build muscles and keep you feeling full. So, go ahead and continue to run, bike, or swim during the Active Phase. If you tend to feel tired or sluggish, maybe you're not eating enough. Make sure to increase your protein and green, leafy vegetable intake.

On the other hand, if you're not exercising when you start the Active Phase, don't worry. We don't expect you to run a mile. You don't have the stamina yet. You can start simply by being more active. Make time to walk fifteen minutes a day. Do it at your own pace, but walk slowly to build up your endurance.

As you lose weight and burn fat by lowering your insulin level, you'll gain more confidence. You'll have more energy to increase your physical activity. Then, you can build up to walking at a brisk pace and increasing the distance. Over time, you can increase the activity to running, swimming, biking, or any other aerobic exercises, including Zumba, dancing, and the more active styles of yoga. Add variations of these exercises, such as aqua Zumba. The key here is to make it fun.

A study published in the journal *Marketing Letters,* in 2014, reveals how your perception and attitudes toward physical activity can affect how much weight you can lose. In the first experiment, fifty-six overweight women were asked to walk on the same one-mile outdoor course for thirty minutes with lunch to follow. Half of the women were told that the walk was for pure pleasure and were given headphones to listen to music during their walk. The other half of the women were told they were exercising and were asked to monitor their exertion. After the mile course, all women were asked to estimate their mood, and the composition of their lunch was compared.

The group of women who were told the walk was exercise ate more calories for lunch, opting for pasta, sugary sodas, and applesauce or chocolate pudding, compared with the group who were told the walk was for pleasure. The former group also reported feeling grumpier and more fatigued compared with the latter group.

A second experiment was conducted to see if similar results could be replicated. Using the same study design, two new groups (some including men) participated, except at the end, all the participants were allowed to fill their own plastic bag with M&M's® as a "thank you." Not surprisingly, the participants who thought they were exercising filled in twice as much candy compared with the participants who thought they were walking for pleasure.

The last experiment took the researchers to the finish line of a marathon relay race where 231 participants between the ages of sixteen to sixty-seven had completed laps of 5 to 10 kilometers. The runners were asked to see if they had enjoyed their race experience. They were offered a choice of a chocolate bar or a cereal bar in consideration for their help. Guess who chose the chocolate bar? The runners who reported the race to be difficult or unsatisfying were more likely to pick the chocolate bar, while the runners who said that they had fun were more likely to choose the cereal bar.

You can see how powerful the mind is. How you perceive physical activity can affect what you choose to eat afterward. For this reason, we focus on teaching you how to change your thinking by challenging cognitive distortions and reframing those thoughts. If you find yourself giving excuses as to why you don't have time to walk fifteen minutes a day, you need to make yourself as important as all your other activities. You're worthy of that walk with your friend or loved one. If it's raining outside, you can still have fun working out with the Wii or a DVD. Just don't make your exercise a chore. Look at it as a chance for you to have some time to yourself to choose to do what you want to do.

Brenda, twenty-six, is a proud mother of an eighteen-month-old son. Prior to having her first child, she was able to maintain her thin frame by keeping herself physically active. She enjoyed hiking with her husband. After the birth of her son, she was unable to lose the baby weight. At 5′6″, she weighed 159 pounds. She wasn't comfortable at that weight, especially given she was at a lighter 125 pounds for most of her adult life.

When Brenda started the Thinsulin Program in March 2015, she didn't exercise at all. Even though her brother is a professional trainer, she found different excuses not to exercise. After losing 8 percent of her initial weight (13 pounds weight loss) in the first month, she became more motivated. At first, she found it difficult to get started on the elliptical machine. She found it tedious and boring, so she added Zumba to her exercise regimen. Once she gained some stamina, she found the elliptical exercise to be more enjoyable. She continued to

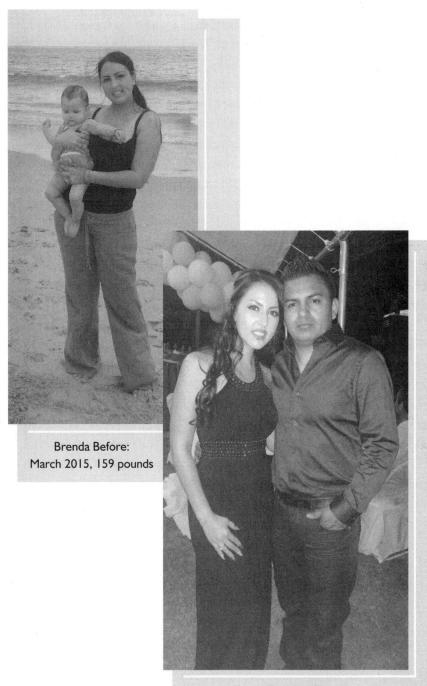

Brenda Before:
March 2015, 159 pounds

Brenda After:
August 2015, 124 pounds

exercise forty-five minutes a day, five days a week. Five months later, she was thrilled to go back down to her comfortable weight of 124 pounds.

Self-monitoring tools can also help to change your behavior and exercise more. Pedometers monitor how many steps you take per day. On average, many people take 3,000 steps per day. It's recommended that you take roughly 10,000 steps per day in order to burn off extra calories. While pedometers are relatively inexpensive, they don't record how hard, long, or often the movement occurs. Accelerometers are more expensive, but they measure the frequency, duration, and intensity of your physical activity. However, accelerometers can't measure resistance. If you're doing strength training, only metabolic devices have sophisticated sensors to accurately calculate how many calories are burned during a day. Of course, these devices are much more expensive.

Be careful not to get all caught up in the technology of these self-monitoring tools. While it's nice to know how many calories you're burning, it's easy to fall back into the calories-in, calories-out thinking if you pay too much attention to how many steps you're taking. Exercise needs to be a part of the comprehensive, biopsychosocial approach, not just viewed by itself.

Throughout the Active Phase, you should build up your stamina by increasing your physical activity week by week. By the time you reach the Passive Phase, you should be doing some form of cardio exercise for at least thirty minutes three times per week.

Chapter 9

CHANGE YOUR THINKING

"Give a man a fish, and you feed him for a day;
teach a man to fish, and you feed him for a lifetime."
—MAIMONIDES

As physicians, we continue to watch how the weight-loss industry promotes meal-replacement shakes, prepackaged meals, appetite suppressants, and calorie-counting as a means to lose weight.
These programs won't work long-term because they're a short-term
solution. Unless weight-loss programs teach you "how to fish," you
won't learn how to overcome the weight-loss plateau and keep the
weight off. You will often be stuck at a certain weight for a period
of time before you gain back the weight. You've probably seen this
"yo-yo" effect with your family members, friends, or even yourself.
How do we break this phenomenon?

In the past, we've spent countless hours educating our patients
in our practice about the USDA food pyramid, and the benefits of a
balanced diet. Despite our thoroughness, we didn't find success with
this approach. Everything we said didn't seem to stick, because we
weren't *teaching* our patients. We were just *telling* our patients what
they could eat based on a list of foods or a set of menus. Telling was
similar to giving our patients a fish rather than teaching them how
to fish.

The Thinsulin Program is a program derived from scientific principles that teaches you how to apply *biological* principles of insulin to burn fat and lose weight—but also *psychological* principles of cognitive behavioral therapy (CBT) to change your thinking; and *social* behavioral techniques to break bad habits. In other words, the Thinsulin Program harnesses the power of three principles—biological, psychological, and social—or biopsychosocial, to ultimately change your eating behavior by changing the way you see food and weight loss and by teaching you to think in terms of insulin. This is so important to successfully fight obesity.

One can't just rely on information alone without understanding underlying concepts. Take, for example, the public education on posting calories. New York City became the first city in the country to require calorie posting at fast-food restaurants in July 2008. The reason was—and is—simple. If customers know how many calories are in an order, perhaps they might choose something healthier or lower in calories. A study conducted by several professors from New York University and Yale tracked customers in poor neighborhoods of New York City with a large poor minority population and high proportion of obesity and diabetes. Customers in these neighborhoods were tracked by what they ordered at McDonald's, Wendy's, Burger King, and Kentucky Fried Chicken and compared them with customers in neighboring Newark, New Jersey, where the calorie posting law isn't in effect. The study reported 50 percent of the customers in New York City noticed the calorie posting. Of the 50 percent who noticed the posting, about 28 percent said the information had influenced the way they ordered. However, when the researchers checked their receipts afterward, they found that orders increased from 825 calories two weeks before the law took effect to 846 calories four weeks after the law was in effect among customers in New York City.

It's not that the calorie posting didn't work—people know that fast foods and sodas are high in calories. It's just that it takes more than nutritional education such as posting calories or reading labels to change eating habits.

Let's look at another example. In spite of doctors' repeated education on the importance of taking antibiotics every day for an upper respiratory infection, there's still a great chance that patients will miss taking their medications during the course of treatment. The rate of noncompliance is high. A study done by Dr. P. Kardas looking at more than thirty thousand patients reported a noncompliance rate of 37.8 percent with antibiotics.

Education alone doesn't change habits. When you focus on details rather than on concepts, there's no way you can cover every aspect. For example, if you're studying for a math test, you're more likely to do better on the test if you master the concepts rather than memorizing the individual problems. If the teacher throws a curveball during the test, you're more likely to extrapolate from your understanding of the concepts to deduct the correct answer. If you only memorize the finer details, you'll be completely lost on the exam.

Likewise, when you master the concept of how foods affect insulin response, and how insulin affects the body, you're more likely to be able to extrapolate from that understanding to select foods that won't spike your insulin level. You won't be hampered by eating the same foods or patronizing the same restaurants daily. If you follow a particular diet or menu, you may run into situations where you won't have access to your type of foods. Then what? Because you only learned the specifics rather than the concepts, you won't be able to adjust to the situation. This will lead to failure as you'll end up eating sweets or carbohydrates. You may feel guilty, leading you to punish yourself by starving the next few days. When you do well, you would then reward yourself, thus repeating the monstrous cycle.

Let's examine what you've learned so far about the biology of weight loss. You've learned that insulin is an important hormone to help you burn fat in the Active Phase. As a result, you've learned how to apply that knowledge to choosing foods that lower insulin level. In the Passive Phase, you'll learn about the science behind the weight-loss plateau and how to overcome it so that you can either maintain your new weight, or lose even more.

As you can see, having a strong understanding of the biology of weight loss provides you with a sound foundation to achieve your goals. But to make even *better* food choices, you also need to change your way of thinking about food and weight loss. By using an effective psychotherapy modality called CBT (cognitive behavioral therapy), you can retrain your brain to think differently about food and weight loss.

If you want to maintain your weight and not "yo yo" up and down, you need to address the social environment temptations and change your bad eating habits. By using behavioral modification, you'll learn to control your cravings and acquire skills to develop healthy eating habits. (We'll talk more about this in Chapter 14, Breaking Bad Habits.)

COGNITIVE BEHAVIORAL THERAPY

Let's talk in more detail about CBT. Psychiatrist Aaron T. Beck developed CBT back in the 1960s, and its primary concept is that thoughts and feelings play a fundamental role in behavior. How does practicing this method help change the way you think?

You have unique experiences that shape you as a person. These life experiences determine your core beliefs. Negative core beliefs will affect how you act and feel because your mind is very powerful. It can send you spiraling down into depression. If you think something often enough, you begin to believe it's true.

Steve, a soft-spoken, forty-five-year-old accountant, was experiencing depression. Recently, he applied for a promotion in his firm. He wanted the new position very much. The promotion, however, went to a coworker who had more experience. Because Steve carried a core belief that "the world is a bad place," he believed that his coworker had an ulterior motive even when that coworker was trying to be nice. In addition, Steve had "all-or-nothing" thinking, characterized by absolute terms such as *never, always,* or *forever.* He felt that he was *always* a failure. He believed that he would *never* be promoted. As a result, Steve felt even more depressed after he was passed over for the promotion.

Steve decided to seek individual therapy for his depression. His therapist decided to use CBT as a treatment. The first goal for Steve was to learn how to identify destructive thoughts and feelings that contributed to the maladaptive behaviors. In his case, Steve identified that the belief that his coworkers are bad people led him to think they had ulterior motives. As a result, he didn't want to work with them.

Next, the therapist helped Steve learn to change how he interprets these destructive thoughts. Steve would challenge these faulty thoughts by examining evidence that supports or doesn't support these negative thoughts. After weighing the evidence, he realized that it didn't support the negative thoughts. This realization challenged his negativity, leading to a cascade of changes that affected his behavior. He no longer believed his coworkers were trying to harm him, and he became more likely to work with them in future projects.

In addition, Steve needed to challenge his all-or-nothing thinking. It's the most common type of negative thinking that represents a major obstacle to self-change. Steve's all-or-nothing thinking trapped him in his own unrealistic standards of being perfect, making it impossible for him to have the energy to make changes in his life. Rather than taking small steps, Steve felt stuck, causing him to have more depression and anxiety.

To help Steve, the therapist focused on Steve's behaviors that were contributing to his difficulties. By identifying destructive thought patterns and changing how he interprets those thoughts, Steve learned to find new ways to change. Instead of waiting to take one giant leap, he took smaller, incremental steps to change his behavior.

Similarly, you may often encounter cognitive distortions about weight loss that affect your feelings and behaviors. How many times have you heard, "If you want to lose weight, just eat less and exercise more?" You've heard it so many times that you believe this must be an undeniable, universal fact. Yet, you've tried eating less, sometimes even starving yourself, without success. You diligently went to the gym, sweating it out on treadmills, but you can't seem to lose any weight. If this was a true statement, why aren't you losing weight?

You begin to believe the problem must be you. You wonder if you lack determination or if you're emotionally weak. You wonder if you're trying hard enough or if maybe you're just not motivated. You grow more frustrated and discouraged.

The truth of the matter is, *nobody* wants to be overweight or obese! This is certainly not your choice. That statement often places the blame squarely on you for the weight gain.

Your desire for weight loss hasn't changed. You want a healthier life. You want more energy to play with your kids. You want to feel more attractive and improve your sex life. You want to prove to yourself that you have self-control. Yet, you're burdened by a conflict between your desire to lose weight and the reality of being unable to do so. The mere thought of lack of control stresses you out. And when you're stressed out from everyday life events, you might turn to ice cream or cake for comfort, only to feel guilty after gorging on sugar. It's a brutal cycle that occurs over and over again—losing weight, regaining it, and then starting the cycle again. This is why so many people fail when they try to lose weight. *It doesn't have to be this way!*

By using CBT, you can challenge this negative thinking and change your behavior. Just like simply telling people to "think positive" if they want to be happy won't work, telling people to eat less and exercise more won't in and of itself lead to weight loss. CBT helps you to successfully make the behavioral change.

The first step of CBT is to *identify* faulty thoughts that contribute to maladaptive behaviors. Let's examine the *"You have to eat less to lose weight"* statement further. At face value, you'd assume that you would lose weight if you ate less—say, only 500 calories a day. What if you only eat ice cream that totals 500 calories per day? Yes, you would be able to lose weight initially but it's terribly unhealthy and completely unsustainable over time. You'll end up eating more to fulfill your hunger. You see, that statement has inherent flaws that may lead you down the wrong path.

OK. No junk food. That's obvious. So, let's say you choose to eat healthfully and restrict your total caloric intake. You should lose weight, correct? What if you eat potatoes, corn, beets, watermelon, pineapple, or bananas? They're all fruits and vegetables that are considered healthy. So, would you lose weight? No, because these high-GI foods are high in sugar content. If you challenge this faulty thinking, you see that thinking in vague terms of "eating less" or "eating healthy" may not guide you in the right direction.

So, how do you *change* your interpretation of this faulty thinking of eating less or eating healthy? What's the root of weight loss? *Lowering insulin.* If you change your thinking from eating less to lowering insulin for weight loss, you can weigh the evidence in terms of spiking insulin or not. You don't need to ask if the foods are high in calories or not, or seem good or bad, or healthy or not.

You simply see the foods in terms of insulin. Do the foods spike insulin or not? If it spikes your insulin level, your body will store fat. If it doesn't, your body will burn fat. This is a scientific fact! By keeping it scientific, it removes a lot of the emotions associated with good or bad, right or wrong, and all-or-nothing thinking. Remember, the all-or-nothing thinking is the most common type of negative thinking that's holding you back. It's the obstacle that prevents you from changing your behavior.

By breaking down the foods you want to eat into five groups and seeing them in terms of insulin, this technique helps you take small, incremental steps to change how you eat, day by day, meal by meal, snack by snack. You no longer have to see weight loss as some giant step that you need to overcome. That's way too intimidating! You don't have negative emotions attached to your actions. That's too discouraging! At each meal, you're breaking down what you're eating into sweets, grains, fruits, vegetables, or proteins. Then, you ask if the foods spike your insulin or not. All you're doing is simply thinking in terms of insulin. After a short period of time, you're able to scan what you're eating and know exactly what will spike your insulin level or not.

Shelly, forty-six, is an energetic woman who came into Lorphen Medical with her husband, Dennis. Her weight of 188 pounds was a bit heavy for her 5'8" frame. She confided that she felt more comfortable at 140 pounds. Due to stress from her work in the insurance business, she gained most of the weight in the past few years. During our first encounter, Shelly was very intrigued with the science of insulin, but she became disengaged when we started talking about sweets. She had this blank stare in total disbelief as she muttered, "You mean I have to give up sweets? I'll *never* be able to give up sugar in my coffee."

Absolute words like *never* are a dead giveaway for the all-or-nothing, negative thinking. In order to change this thinking, it's important to help Shelly understand that this statement is problematic. Yet, if confronted too strongly and without empathy, Shelly may be pushed away further. So I first acknowledged that drinking black coffee may not be as good, and then asked her in a supportive tone, "Is it a bit too strong to say that you'll never be able to give up sugar in your coffee?" By challenging this all-or-nothing thinking, Shelly admitted that she could do it, but she didn't want to because "black coffee is disgusting."

The fact that Shelly admitted that she could do it, but she chose not to, was quite significant! There's room for her to change now as her thinking moved from "never" to a choice.

Next, I asked, "What's your goal?"

She said she wants to lose weight and be healthier.

I pushed some more. "Wouldn't it be nice for you to burn off all that fat?"

"Yes, that would be awesome," she replied. "That's what I want."

"What happens when you spike your insulin level?"

"Your body stores fat," she said.

"Does sugar spike insulin level?"

"Most definitely!" she said, with much more confidence than she had in the beginning.

Now that Shelly was able to link the sugar in her coffee to spiking her insulin level, she had a choice to make. If she wanted to reach her goal, she would have to lower her insulin level. Maybe that meant she had to drink it black.

As you can see from this exchange, there wasn't any mention of what's "good" or "bad," "right" or "wrong." These are emotionally charged, arbitrary words that often come with the territory of dieting.

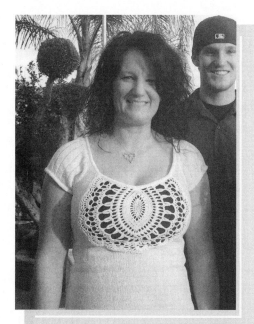

Shelly Before: March 2013, 188 pounds

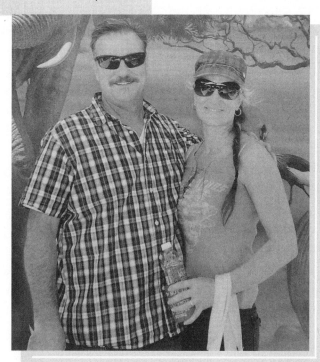

Shelly After:
November 2013, 142 pounds

Why would sugar in your coffee be "bad" or "wrong"? In fact, having sugar in your coffee actually makes the coffee taste "good." You see, these words have so many different meanings to people, it is distracting them from what's most important: lowering insulin.

Shelly's journey helped her achieve her goal weight of 142 pounds after eight months. "I don't like counting carbs," she shared. "Thinsulin is conceptually easier to follow because it teaches you the science. I look at food differently now."

As you transition to the Passive Phase, CBT will be used to challenge more cognitive distortions that may impede your progress in your journey for weight loss. We'll address these cognitive distortions when we get to the Passive Phase chapter.

You may ask, "If I'm burning fat by lowering insulin, why can't I just stay in the Active Phase?" Unfortunately, your body will fight against the weight loss as defense for your survival. Your body will win and you'll hit the weight-loss plateau, which separates the two phases. You simply can't fight your own biology, and you'll enter the Passive Phase. Your goal shifts to increasing your insulin level while maintaining your weight for the next three months.

If you need to lose more weight after you've undergone the Passive Phase, you can go back to the Active Phase and lower your insulin level again in order to burn fat. You will learn in Chapter 10 why you need to increase your insulin level during the Passive Phase in order to overcome the weight-loss plateau.

If you're happy with your weight, you'll shift your goals to maintaining your weight by focusing more on the psychological and behavioral issues that may derail your journey. By using CBT and behavioral modifications, you'll learn new skills to help you avoid the pitfalls that put you at risk for weight regain.

Throughout this journey, you'll learn a lot about concepts ranging from the biology of insulin to the psychology of CBT. While it's important to learn "how to fish," what you'll learn the most about is you.

THINSULIN
ACTIVE PHASE MILESTONES
Weeks 1–16

Eat five times per day.

- Breakfast: 1 portion of dairy product (only at breakfast), protein meat or seafood, or egg white
- Morning snack: 1 portion of fresh, low-GI fruit (apple, orange, grapes, or berries)
- Lunch: at least 1 portion of green, leafy vegetables and at least 1 portion of protein meat or seafood
- Afternoon snack: 1 portion of raw nuts
- Dinner: at least 1 portion of green, leafy vegetables and at least 1 portion of protein meat or seafood

Break down your foods into 5 categories.

- Sweets: desserts, snacks, and sugary drinks (water, unsweetened iced tea, and unsweetened coffee will not spike insulin)
- Grains: even healthy grains will spike the insulin level
- Vegetables: "Potatoes, corn, carrots and beets, these are the veggies I cannot eat."
- Fruits: apple, orange, grapes, or berries (cherries, strawberries, cranberries, blackberries, raspberries, and blueberries)
- Proteins: egg whites, chicken, turkey, beef, pork, fish, or seafood

Once you've grouped them, ask yourself if the foods will spike insulin. Use the traffic light analogy.

- Red Light: STOP! These food groups will spike your insulin level. Don't eat sweets, grains, and starchy vegetables.
- Yellow Light: BE CAUTIOUS. These foods may spike your insulin level if you eat more than one portion. That's why you can only have a handful of nuts in the afternoon and one total portion of fresh fruit in the morning.
- Green Light: GO. These foods will not spike your insulin level, so you can eat as much as you want at breakfast, lunch, or dinner. Make sure you have at least one portion of protein meat and one portion of green, leafy vegetables for lunch and dinner.

WEEK 2

Weigh yourself at the start of week two. If you didn't lose between 3 to 5 pounds, you're still eating foods that spike your insulin level.

- Create a food log. Write down everything you eat for breakfast, snack, lunch, snack, and dinner.
- On the same food log, break down the foods into 5 categories. The difference here is that you're writing it down rather than just visually looking at it.
- Use the traffic light analogy to see if the foods will spike your insulin level.

Begin to walk fifteen minutes a day along with thinking in terms of insulin. It should get easier by week two.

WEEK 3

Weigh yourself at the start of Week three. Again, if you're still not losing between 3 and 5 pounds, there's something you're doing that is keeping your insulin elevated.

Take a picture of all your food and drink intake for breakfast, snack, lunch, snack, and dinner.

Text the pictures to someone who has gone through Thinsulin. Get creative. Maybe post it online. Someone will help guide you to choose foods that won't spike your insulin level. Post your questions on Facebook (www.facebook.com/thinsulin).

WEEK 4

Continue to break down the foods into 5 categories. Make sure to use the traffic light analogy to see what foods spike your insulin level.

WEEKS 5–8

"I'm not on a diet! I'm doing Thinsulin." If you're lowering your insulin level correctly, you should drop at least 5 percent of your body weight. By now, friends and family members will begin to ask you what you're doing. Avoid using the word "diet" and teach them about Thinsulin. Continue to break down the foods into 5 groups and think in terms of insulin.

WEEKS 9–12

Remember, "weight loss is a journey, not a destination!" It's easy to deviate from Thinsulin two months after you start.

1. Don't be surprised if you didn't lose weight if you cheated. Remember that it takes three weeks to lower the insulin level again once you cheat. Don't blame yourself for "being bad"! That's the old way of thinking. You understand that weight loss is a journey. Just accept the fact and move on. Figure out what you did and why it happened.

If you cheated because you're hungry or craving sweets, look back at what you ate for lunch or dinner. Maybe you have to eat more protein and green, leafy vegetables to keep you full.

If you cheated because you skipped meals earlier in the day, stop for a second and ask yourself if your health is as important as your work, family, or friends? You're important enough to have fifteen minutes to plan your meals ahead of time so that you don't have to skip meals.

2. Are you bored of eating the same foods? If you are, then mix it up. Find new recipes and challenge yourself to find foods that won't spike your insulin level. You're not on a diet, so you don't need to suffer.

3. Make sure you're still physically active. Increase from walking fifteen minutes to an activity that will increase your heart rate so that you can build up some endurance.

WEEKS 13–16

Get ready to overcome the weight-loss plateau. You haven't hit the plateau yet—that usually starts around four months—but it's important to review this chapter again. You need to understand that in a few weeks, your body will win and you'll hit the weight-loss plateau. No matter how hard you try, your weight will stay relatively the same. It's important to accept this fact or you'll set yourself up for disappointment. It's simply unrealistic to lose the same amount of weight you lost in the first few months. Be prepared. The good news is, you're going to be able to reintroduce grains and starchy vegetables once you hit the plateau and enter the Passive Phase.

PART IV

THINSULIN
PHASE TWO:
THE PASSIVE PHASE

Scott, thirty-three, is a 6'2" firefighter who lives with his family in California. In October 2014, his massive weight of 318 had placed his health and his job in serious jeopardy. As a firefighter, he knew he could place others' lives in harm's way if he made just one wrong move during the physical requirements of his job.

"Firefighters must be in great shape for responding to unknown calls," said Scott. "What if something happened that was beyond my abilities—like, I got a call for a big brushfire? I wasn't prepared. Knowing that was extremely stressful."

Stress, Scott was soon to discover, was the state that triggered his steady climb from 280 pounds in early 2014 to his ultimate high of 318 when he hit his psychological bottom that October.

Ironically, Scott's weight creeped up just as he experienced the joy of familial life changes: his wife birthed their first baby; they bought their first house; he took family leave and stayed home to raise their son. As amazing as these events were, the stress of them triggered Scott's first real bout of out-of-control eating. He began to isolate, and his chronic food bingeing and lack of physicality eroded his self-esteem.

As his weight climbed toward the 300-pound mark, one day in September Scott had an epiphany. He realized that his weight gain would keep him from doing what he had loved best as a child—riding bikes and surfing. These were two sports he had grown up playing with his dad. "My call to action was to be there for my son," Scott explained. "I had fallen in love with him and I wanted to be active—bike with him and more as my dad had done with me." Scott had also loved being a bodybuilder, jogger, and weightlifter.

Scott got fitness-tested once a year for his job as a firefighter. He had missed the test the previous year, and asked for and got a deferral, but the new test was imminent. "I was so out of shape that I wouldn't have met the minimum treadmill requirements."

With his job at risk and unable to imagine a future in which he couldn't play with his son, Scott's back was against the wall when he walked into the Lorphen Medical Clinic that fall. He knew he had gained weight, but he had no idea it had crept up to such a very serious and life-threatening weight.

Every year, millions of Americans make New Year's resolutions to lose weight. Right before summer, millions more go on a diet as they get ready for fun in the sun. They latch on to any new gimmick just to have a chance to fit in their bikini again. These Americans, like Scott, are not short on motivation, but they often lack the knowledge to lose weight.

In order for Scott to succeed, he needed to learn more about the science of insulin and its effect on fat metabolism. He didn't know that if he cheated, it would take three weeks to lower his insulin again. No wonder he wasn't able to lose weight before! He asked questions. He wanted to absorb as much information as possible. He soon mastered the simple technique of breaking down food into five groups. He remembered the traffic light analogy, avoiding the red, being cautious on the yellow, and eating as much as he wanted on the green.

Scott knew Thinsulin was for him. He dropped 30 pounds in the first month despite going on a family cruise one week after starting the program. After two months, he lost a total of 50 pounds. That's almost a pound a day. He was eating five times a day. He never felt hungry like when he was on other diet programs.

He also realized that stress had been his kryptonite, and losing weight had been a panacea: it lowered his blood pressure, got him in shape for his job, and helped him feel more in control of his life. It was the combination of learning the science of Thinsulin to go along with his motivation that helped Scott stay on track.

Scott utilized the behavioral principles embedded in Thinsulin to break his bad habits. He set up an online account for his family and began posting daily shots of his weight scale to show that he's committed. He also posts his workout and even photos of his salad!

He has learned to troubleshoot. "I wasn't disciplined at work," he explained. "When I get off a twenty-four-hour shift, I'm tired.

I needed to keep more greens and proteins on hand. Stay full. Pack stuff and cook beforehand—and the payoff is that I'm in the best shape of my life!"

He understood that the weight loss would slow down as the body naturally attempts to maintain homeostasis. By the time he hit the weight-loss plateau, he had lost 80 pounds, about 25 percent of his initial weight. He was anxious to lose more weight, but he knew his insulin level couldn't stay low forever.

In the Passive Phase, the goal shifts from lowering insulin and losing weight (the Active Phase) to carefully increasing insulin and maintaining the weight loss. This enables you to overcome the plateau and later go back to the Active Phase to lose even more weight.

Scott shifted gears and entered the Passive Phase. He was cautious at first to have an enjoyment food after his meal. He was afraid of gaining back all his weight if he had that one slice of bread. He had worked so hard to get to this point, and he certainly didn't want to blow it.

Despite his amazing progress, he still had remnants of his old thinking. He pondered how many calories were in the slice of bread rather than its effect on insulin. But eating that one slice of bread served the purpose of increasing his insulin level without leading to a disastrous outcome. He merely needed to have only one enjoyment food at breakfast, lunch, or dinner.

He was relieved to know that adding back bread or rice to his meals didn't cause weight gain. It didn't cause weight loss either, but the goal in this phase was to maintain his weight. He needed to increase the insulin level so that when his body resets in three months, it would be much easier for him to go back to the Active Phase and drop the elevated insulin again. That time would come. All he had to do was maintain his weight and slowly increase his enjoyment food to two total portions a day.

Scott also kept up with his exercise, cycling about 20 to 30 miles three times a week. He got back into swimming. He stayed active while focusing on eating five times a day and thinking in terms of insulin. When he wanted dessert, he would make sure that he didn't eat any other enjoyment food that day. That sweet represented two enjoyments for the day. Sometimes, he didn't think a cookie was worth giving up oatmeal or spaghetti.

After three months on the Passive Phase, he went back to the Active Phase. He kept up with his exercise and saw more fat and weight come off. By now, he was a seasoned pro at maintaining his newfound freedom. He could go to birthday parties, vacations, buffets, or fine restaurants without fear of gaining weight. He knew he just needed to think in terms of insulin.

Scott continued to lose weight. As of October 2015, he had lost 115 pounds, and now weighed close to 200 pounds. His success piqued the interest of his coworkers, friends, and family, who all wanted to learn more about Thinsulin.

Chapter 10

OVERCOMING THE WEIGHT-LOSS PLATEAU

Thousands of diet book authors claim to have revealed secrets to weight loss. Yet diets themselves are often too confusing to figure out. Advertisers have tried to simplify diets to their basic core. If you prefer high fat and high protein without fruits, you might have tried the Atkins or South Beach diets. If you like whole grains and lots of fruits and vegetables, maybe you've checked out the Mediterranean diet. Perhaps you've crossed paths with the anti-inflammatory Zone diet developed by Dr. Barry Sears. If a simple smoothie for breakfast or lunch wets your whistle, you might have tried the Slim-Fast or Herbalife shakes. If packaged meals make dieting more bearable, maybe you've signed up for Jenny Craig, NutriSystem, or Weight Watchers.

By restricting your caloric intake, you can lose weight on any of these diets, but the hard part is keeping the weight off long term. It's easy to start a diet, but it's difficult to maintain the same diet plan over the long haul. In addition, you may lose weight in the beginning only to find yourself stuck at that weight no matter how hard you try. In fact, there comes a point in every diet in which the body can no longer lose weight regardless of what you eat or how much you exercise. This is what we call the "weight-loss plateau." In the Thinsulin

Program, it typically occurs around four months, and marks the start of the Passive Phase. We'll show you how to overcome this dreaded plateau. But first, we'll help you understand the biological reasons for it.

After losing weight during the four-month Active Phase, your body will eventually reach what doctors call "homeostasis." It's the dynamic state of stability between the environment and our bodies through a complex balance involving the nervous, endocrine, respiratory, and circulatory systems. All systems work together to maintain energy stability.

Think of it like a thermostat. When the temperature in a heated room reaches the set limit, the heating unit switches off, and the temperature falls. Then, when the temperature drops to a lower limit, the heating unit switches on again. Within this range, the thermostat maintains a steady room temperature.

Similarly, our bodies' natural systems work to maintain our weight within a specific range by keeping our sugar and electrolytes level and the body temperature at a constant, balanced range. You see a lot of weight loss in the first few months, but over time the rate of weight loss dwindles. This is your body's attempt to maintain homeostasis. Even if you ate the exact same foods as you did in the beginning, you still won't lose weight. You've hit the dreaded weight-loss plateau. But wait—why would your body want to maintain homeostasis and stop you from losing weight? Doesn't your body know that you need to lose more weight in order to reduce other cardiovascular risk factors?

Unfortunately, your body doesn't know that you're intentionally trying to lose weight. Your body sees the weight loss as a form of starvation arising from a possible famine due to a flood or drought. Through human evolution, your body boasts a built-in protective mechanism called "adaptive thermogenesis" to protect you from starvation by fighting against weight loss. Researchers have shown that weight loss results in biological adaptations, specifically a decline in energy expenditure and an increase in hunger, both of which promote weight regain. In other words, your body wants to regain the weight it has lost by reducing the energy you burn and increasing your food craving and preference for calorically dense foods. There's simply no avoiding it. Our bodies evolved to keep weight on us and to store food as fat in case our food supply dwindles and we face the future risk of starvation. It's only a matter of time after you've started your weight-loss program before you hit the weight-loss plateau.

How long does it take to bump up against the weight-loss plateau? If you look at the dynamic energy balance models that scientists have done to accurately predict weight change, they have shown that it takes between one to two years. However, research studies showed that weight loss typically stabilizes at six months or sooner. Why is there a discrepancy? A study published in the *American Journal of Clinical Nutrition* showed that the plateau occurred earlier because of an intermittent lack of diet adherence rather than metabolic adaptation. Simply stated, if you're cheating and still spiking your insulin level during the Active Phase, you'll hit the plateau sooner. In our clinical experience, we've observed that our patients tend to reach the weight-loss plateau after roughly four months.

What do you do once you reach the weight-loss plateau? The current advice from some nutritionists is to eat even less and exercise even more in order to create an energy deficit. In theory, this will force your body to burn its fat storage in order for you to overcome the plateau. But in practice, is it really possible for you to eat less than what you were eating while you were in the Active Phase? Very unlikely! Keep in mind that your body's biological response pressures your body to regain its weight. Over time, you might get discouraged, and even give in to your cravings. You may resort back to your bad eating habits and in no time, you'll gain back some or all of your weight. Does this sound familiar at all?

To move beyond this biological restraint and fight weight regain, you have to take a different approach. This approach unlocks the door to the Passive Phase. Because homeostasis involves a complex balance, you need to respond with your own carefully controlled counterbalance. We've discovered a way to manipulate the body's natural rhythms to overcome the weight-loss plateau. While most weight-loss programs teach you how to reduce your total energy stores, we'll teach you how to beat the weight-loss plateau by changing your insulin level.

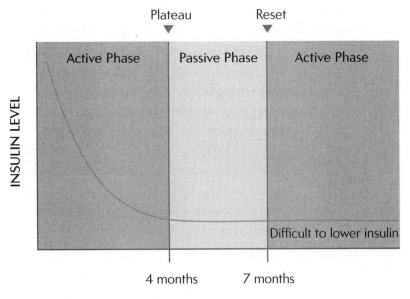

Figure 13 Overview of Active and Passive Phase diagram

OVERVIEW OF ACTIVE AND PASSIVE PHASE

Let's look at the Overview diagram. You see that during the Active Phase, your insulin level drops until you hit the weight-loss plateau. At that moment, you can't lower your insulin level much more as it also reaches a steady state. When your body resets to allow you to lose weight again, your insulin level is already so low, it's biologically difficult to lower it any more. Therefore, even though your body is ready for you to lose weight, you won't be able to because you're unable to lower your insulin any farther. This means you won't be able to burn fat and lose more pounds.

There's evidence for a set point that regulates your body weight, but we don't know exactly how long the plateau lasts. At some point, your body will "reset" to allow you to lose weight again. If that's not the case, no one would ever lose weight after they hit the weight-loss plateau. In our clinical experience, we've observed that our patients can begin to lose weight again after three months of hitting the plateau.

As you can see, it doesn't make sense for you to keep your insulin level low during the Passive Phase since your body prevents you from losing weight anyway. While you're waiting for your body to reset, your biological drives will make you crave more carbohydrates so that you can regain the weight. But actually, you can eat more carbs to increase your insulin level—within limits—during the Passive Phase and this will allow you to eventually *lose* weight!

Let's look at another diagram below. Let's say you hit the weight-loss plateau. Instead of keeping your insulin low, you slowly and carefully increase your carb intake during the Passive Phase so that your insulin level will rise very gently. Think of it as ascending a roller coaster. At the end of three months, your body resets to allow weight loss again, and you return to the Active Phase and pick up where you

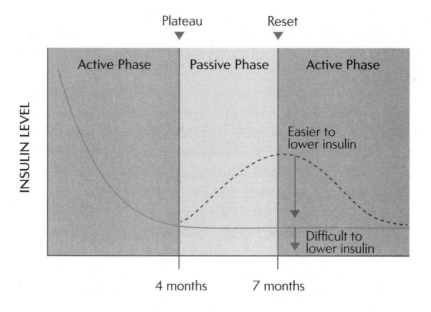

Figure 14 Active and Passive Phase diagram #2

left off. Your insulin level is higher than it was before, so now you can work on lowering it again. In our practice, we've seen people get down to the lowest weight of their adult lives. It's amazing!

Pretty neat, huh? Now you're working with the magic hormone to lose weight and keep it off.

WHY LOW-GI IS BEST

There's another important reason why you can't avoid carbs and sweets forever. What you eat—whether it's low-fat/high-carb; low-glycemic-index; or low-carb—affects the way you use energy. A study published in the *Journal of the American Medical Association* studied the effect of three diets on resting energy expenditure (REE, also known as the *basal metabolic rate*) and total energy expenditure (TEE). REE is the number of calories you would burn if you stayed in bed all day, and TEE is the total calories you would burn in an average day. After participants lost 10 to 15 percent of their weight, they were put on a low-fat, high-glycemic-load diet (60 percent carbohydrates, 20 percent fat, 20 percent protein), low-glycemic-index diet (40 percent carbohydrates, 40 percent fat, 20 percent protein), or a low-carb diet (10 percent carbohydrates, 60 percent fat, and 30 percent protein).

The low-fat, high-glycemic-load diet reduced the REE and TEE the most, putting these participants at the highest risk for weight regain by lowering the number of calories you would burn the most compared with the other two diets in a day. Unfortunately, this is the type of diet conventionally recommended for most people, even though the research showed otherwise. In plain English: don't go on a low-fat diet after you've lost weight.

What if you continue eating a high-protein, low-carb diet? The study showed the low-carb diet reduced the REE and TEE the least, so the body can burn more calories in a day than when practicing the other two diets. However, the low-carb diet increased cortisol secretion, which promoted more fat deposits, insulin resistance, and cardiovascular disease. Cortisol is a steroid hormone produced by the adrenal glands in response to stress. Cortisol mobilizes triglycerides from storage and relocates them to visceral fat cells. In other words, the fat goes straight to the belly and is hard to shed. Even though you can lose some weight, continuing the low-carb diet will increase the risk for insulin resistance. You don't want to continue keeping your insulin level low with a low-carb diet after you've lost weight.

The low-glycemic-index diet had similar, although smaller metabolic benefits but without the harmful effects. The study concluded that this strategy, which reduces glycemic load rather than dietary fat, is superior for weight-loss maintenance and cardiovascular health. Put differently, a low-GI diet is best after you've lost weight and hit the plateau because it will increase your insulin level slowly over time without causing daily spikes.

RAISING YOUR INSULIN WISELY

The concept is simple, but the practice, like most new habits, requires diligence. If you haven't changed your eating habits, you run the risk of regaining the weight when you reintroduce carbs and sweets during the Passive Phase. This is why it's critical to reintroduce them in a controlled manner. It's equally critical that you eat them at breakfast, lunch, or dinner only. You have to continue with fruit as a morning snack and a handful of nuts as your afternoon snack.

The simple yet crucial act of thinking in terms of insulin will guide you through the journey. You've had four months to maximize your weight loss by lowering your insulin level before you arrived at the plateau. To overcome it, you need to do exactly the opposite. You'll still eat five meals a day, except now you can add the foods that you avoided during the Active Phase to breakfast, lunch, or dinner.

Let's say after four months of success in the Active Phase, you're craving a burger for lunch. Prior to working the Thinsulin Program, you may have eaten a burger with fries and sipped your favorite soda. From the study described, you understand that if you eat high-carbs like this, you'll regain your weight in no time. However, you can still maintain your weight and enjoy your meal. Instead, you can choose only *one* portion of the food that may spike your insulin level. In other words, if you decide to eat the hamburger with the buns (grains), then don't have the fries (starchy vegetables) or soda (sweets). If you really want to eat the fries, then avoid eating the hamburger bun and elect a lettuce-wrapped burger instead. The idea here is to choose only one portion per day of your enjoyment food in order to minimize the insulin spike. You'll learn more in the next chapter, "How to Eat Carbs Without Gaining Weight."

In short, at first it can be very demoralizing when you hit the weight-loss plateau. You're confused because you don't know why you can't seem to lose any more weight, even though you've changed the way you eat. You wonder if you're doing something wrong. Instead, you can turn it all around with one simple act. You guessed it—by thinking in terms of insulin! By changing your thinking, you can overcome the weight-loss plateau.

Depending on which phase you're in, you're always either raising or lowering your insulin. In the Active Phase, your goal is to maximize the weight loss by lowering your insulin level. On the other hand, during the Passive Phase, your goal shifts to maintaining your weight and increasing your insulin level in order for you to overcome the plateau. Once your insulin rises and your body is ready for you to lose weight again, you can shift back to the Active Phase and lower your insulin level—and drop pounds—once again.

We presented our research at The Obesity Society's 33rd Annual Scientific Meeting Poster Session during ObesityWeek 2015. This small observational study over one year showed that ten patients lost an average of 16.6 percent of baseline body weight at the end of the Active Phase, gained back 1.1 percent at the end of the Passive Phase, and lost 6.7 percent of their body weight after a second round of the Active Phase. Their BMI dropped from 38 to 29.8 over the course of the study, taking them from being severely obese to overweight.

Chapter 11

HOW TO EAT CARBS WITHOUT GAINING WEIGHT

When our patients hear that they need to raise their insulin level in the Passive Phase, they often have reservations. They like the idea of expanding their food choices, but they're afraid of weight gain if they eat rice or potatoes again. They tell us that by now, they're so used to staying away from foods that would spike their insulin level that it seems counterintuitive to eat grains or starchy vegetables again. They have undergone quite a compelling transformation since they started the Active Phase four months ago, when they wondered—and often seriously questioned—if they could actually stop eating desserts, sodas, and grains. Now, as they carry out the Passive Phase, not only is it easy for them to keep their insulin low, but they often don't want to begin eating grains or starchy vegetables again.

This is why it's so important to understand the science. In the Passive Phase, it's critical to *raise* your insulin level again in order to overcome the weight-loss plateau. With Thinsulin, you'll use the natural rhythms of your body to either lose or maintain your weight, depending what phase you're in.

This chapter focuses on how to reintroduce grains and starchy vegetables in your meals *without* weight gain.

REINTRODUCING CARBS

The Passive Phase lasts for three months. During this time, you'll need to reintroduce carbs slowly or you'll develop intense cravings that will overcome your self-control—leading you to eat too many carbs. That's why you don't want to add back sweets in the first month. It's too soon and it'll only set you up for possible failure. Instead, you'll stick with grains, starchy vegetables, or high-GI fruits. We refer to the carbs that you'll reintroduce during this phase as "enjoyment food." The idea is simple. You'll slowly increase the portion of your enjoyment food in a controlled manner so that your insulin level goes up but not your weight. You may have your enjoyment food at breakfast, lunch, or dinner. For example, you may have fries (starchy vegetables) or hamburger buns (grains) for lunch. The enjoyment food cannot replace your morning or afternoon snack. Let's look at the chart.

Number of Weeks	Carbs Portion Size (generally, the size of a fist)
Weeks 17–18	½ portion at breakfast, lunch, or dinner. No sweets as desserts, snacks, and drinks.
Weeks 19–20	1 portion at breakfast, lunch, or dinner. No sweets as desserts, snacks, and drinks.
Weeks 21–22	½ portion at breakfast, lunch, or dinner. 1 portion at breakfast, lunch, or dinner. 1 portion of sweets as a dessert, snack, or drink. (Sweets are equivalent to 2 portions per day of grains, starchy vegetables, or high-GI fruits. Sweets are *not* to be used in addition to the portions above.)
Weeks 23–28	1 portion at breakfast, lunch, or dinner. 1 portion at breakfast, lunch, or dinner. 1 portion of sweets as a dessert, snack, or drink. (Sweets are equivalent to 2 portions per day of grains, starchy vegetables, or high-GI fruits. Sweets are *not* to be used in addition to the portions above.)
Week 29– May enter Active Phase	Lower insulin level.

PASSIVE PHASE
(BEGINS AT MONTH FIVE, WEEK 17)

When you start the Passive Phase, eat only half a portion of the enjoyment food per day for the first two weeks at breakfast, lunch, or dinner. It may be easier to start with eating half a portion of oatmeal for breakfast. This will help you ease back into eating grains again. Remember that one portion is about the size of your fist. You don't have to use a scale to measure out your portion. If you feel more comfortable with a scale, you may use it. That's entirely up to you. What we want to emphasize here is the concept. By limiting the amount of your enjoyment food, you can limit the degree of insulin spiking.

After two weeks of starting the Passive Phase, you can increase your enjoyment food to a full portion for another two weeks. You may not split the portion into different meals. In our experience, we noticed that when our patients split their alloted portions into two separate meals, they tend to underestimate their half portion, and they would often eat more than what they should. For example, at weeks two to four, you can't have a half portion of oatmeal for breakfast and the other half portion of rice for lunch. In short, you're increasing your enjoyment food to a total of one portion by the end of the first month in the Passive Phase.

By your second month in the Passive Phase, at week four to six, you may increase your total of enjoyment food to one and a half portions per day. The one portion and the other half portion must be eaten at separate meals. For example, you may have half a portion of wheat toast for breakfast and one portion of spaghetti for dinner. You may continue to increase your enjoyment food by another one-half portion, for a total of two portions per day from week seven to eight. Again, you must separate the two portions into different meals. You may not have any other enjoyment food if you have sweets. Remember, sweets count as two portions. If you choose to have a sweet as a dessert or drink, make sure to have it at breakfast, lunch, or dinner after you've eaten your vegetables and proteins.

You'll continue to eat two portions of enjoyment food per day in your third month of the Passive Phase. After three months of raising your insulin, you may decide to go back to the Active Phase if you want to lose more weight by lowering your insulin level again. If you're happy with maintaining your weight, you may continue eating two portions of enjoyment food per day. By the end of six weeks, you'll be eating up to two portions of carbs per day.

Now that you know how to slowly increase your portion size of grains, starchy vegetables, or high-GI fruits, we'll review in more detail the food groups that you'll eat during the Passive Phase.

Grains

If you choose to eat anything made out of grains, consider picking low-GI grains, such as wheat, multigrain bread, barley, brown rice, or oatmeal. Another good option is quinoa. Even though you can have grains at breakfast, lunch, or dinner, understand that high-GI grains such as white rice, pasta, noodles, and tortillas will spike your insulin level more than low-GI grains. The spiking of insulin will lead to a rebound effect where you'll get more tired and hungrier. Be aware of this situation. As for cereal for breakfast, don't be fooled by the label boasting how much fortified calcium or how many vitamins it contains. You still need to think in terms of insulin. In this case, you already know that cereal (as a grain) will spike your insulin level. The question is, "How much?" You definitely want to choose cereals without any added sugar. For example, choose plain Cheerios over Honey Nut Cheerios, for obvious reasons. In short, you want to increase your insulin level during the Passive Phase, but you want to minimize that spike by picking low-GI grains over high-GI grains.

Vegetables

Starchy vegetables such as potatoes, corn, carrots, and beets will definitely spike your insulin level. You may have only one portion of the starchy vegetable at breakfast, lunch, or dinner during the Passive

Phase. Just remember that the starchy vegetables are part of your enjoyment food so you can't have grains or high-GI fruits on top of the starchy vegetables. For example, if you decide to eat potato wedges with your lemon and garlic roasted chicken, you can't have some roasted corn because this will tip over your insulin level. You want your insulin level to rise, but you don't want to overdo it either. That's why you can have only one portion of potatoes, corn, carrots, or beets at breakfast, lunch, or dinner. Depending on how far along you are in the Passive Phase, you may have another portion, but at a different meal. Always remember to break down your foods and group them into the five food categories. That's the only way you know how to limit to one portion. Suppose you're eating steamed vegetables. If you individually break down what the steamed vegetables contain, you may see that there are broccoli, carrots, and corn. If you decide to use starchy vegetables as your portion during the Passive Phase, you may choose to eat steamed carrots or corn, but not both. Broccoli doesn't increase the insulin level, so you can have as much of it as you want.

You may have wondered why you need to avoid eating carrots. Some studies report the GI and GL to be 49 and 2, respectively, because the carrots store starch in the roots as resistant starch so it may not spike insulin as rapidly available starch. That's why carrots are allowed in some low-carb diets. However, some sources still list the GI of carrots as 92, making it more likely to spike insulin level. Based on this discrepancy and confusion, we group carrots as part of the root vegetables for simplicity, making it easier for you to remember what foods to avoid.

Now that you have gained more knowledge, you can apply that knowledge and expand your food choices. You notice that peaches and pears have low GI as well. Therefore, you can eat a peach or pear instead of just an apple, orange, grapes, or berries.

Fruits

The morning snack is similar for both the Active and Passive Phases. You may have only one portion of a low-GI fruit, such as an apple, orange, grapes, or berries. If you want to eat a high-GI fruit, such as a pineapple, banana, or watermelon, you may have this enjoyment food at breakfast, lunch, or dinner. These high-GI fruits will spike your insulin, so if you choose to eat watermelon during an afternoon picnic, then you can't have any grains or starchy vegetables. Remember, you're allowed to have only one enjoyment food to increase your insulin level at breakfast, lunch, or dinner. Therefore, you have to decide what you really want. You're not completely depriving yourself of foods. You're just choosing what you really want to eat.

Sweets

As you can guess, having sweets too soon will put you on a collision course for failure. Sweets will make you crave more sweets, and it's a vicious cycle. Yet, it's unrealistic to imagine that you can't have cheesecake for the rest of your life. There must be a balance between the competing forces.

As you're reintroducing grains, starchy vegetables, or high-GI fruits slowly back to your meals, it's not recommended for you to reintroduce sweets as a snack, drink, or dessert until the middle of the second month (after six weeks of the Passive Phase). When you feel that you have better control, the sweets may be added later on. Again, you may add the sweets as your enjoyment food only at breakfast, lunch, or dinner. If you choose any sweets, this will be the only enjoyment food you can have for the entire day. You may not have any grains, starchy vegetables, or high-GI fruits at any other meals. Your sweets are equivalent to two portions per day of grains, starchy vegetables, or high-GI fruits.

You should never eat the sweets as a morning or afternoon snack. Ever! In our experience, we notice this is why so many people fail and regain back a lot of weight. It may be as innocent as having a chocolate chip cookie as a snack one time. But the next time it will be two cookies as a morning snack, and then more sweets later on. Over time, your sweet cravings may intensify to a point where you could lose all control. We've seen this numerous times, not just with our patients, but also in our personal struggles to control our sweet cravings.

If you decide to have a dessert, it's very important to plan your day first. For example, if you decide to eat the best key lime pie in town tomorrow at a dinner party, then you need to make sure that you're not having any other enjoyment foods for breakfast, lunch, or dinner. So at dinner, you may need to avoid the oven-warmed bread, perfectly cooked mashed potatoes, or delicious linguini if you really want that key lime pie. If you decide to eat all the enjoyment foods, you know for sure your pancreas would have to work overtime to bring down the rush of blood glucose. Take a moment to visualize what that would do to your fat storage and weight over time if you didn't exercise any control.

Here's another scenario. What if you attend a noon birthday party and the red velvet cake isn't served until three p.m.? That timing cuts into your afternoon snack of a handful of nuts! You've got a major dilemma here!

The red velvet cake is served two hours after you've finished your lunch. In addition, you didn't know that they were serving your favorite cake, or you wouldn't have eaten oatmeal for breakfast. What do you do? Stick to the rule. Your enjoyment foods can only be consumed at breakfast, lunch, or dinner. You should wrap up that delicious slice of cake to go and eat it the next day if you have to.

Don't "cheat" by bending the rule. If you justify it by saying, "A small bite doesn't contain that many calories so it's OK to eat," then you've reverted back to your old way of thinking that weight loss is about eating less. You must always remember to think in terms of insulin. If you succumb and cheat, what's there to stop you from doing the same thing tomorrow? What about the next day? Pretty soon, everything that you've built up to this point will fall apart. It's not worth it to cheat! You're not depriving yourself if you save the slice of cake for the next day. By being disciplined, you'll grow to feel good about the person in the mirror, too—as the person in the mirror shrinks to a smaller size!

As for sugary drinks, it has taken you months to get rid of the sugar cravings. By reintroducing sugary beverages, those sugar cravings will return with a vengeance. Besides, where would you add the sugary beverages? They don't belong as a snack, meal, or dessert. As a result, they shouldn't be part of the equation. Just stick to water or unsweetened iced tea. But if you absolutely are compelled to drink a soda, juice, or sweetened iced tea, just treat the sugary drink as a sweet. You may have that soda only at breakfast, lunch, or dinner, and that soda represents all your enjoyment food for the day. Ask yourself, "Is it worth it to drink that root beer, or would I rather eat some fries for lunch and a little spaghetti for dinner?" It's up to you. Thinsulin is all about choices.

WHEN TO EAT YOUR CARBS

Is there a particular sequence in which you can have your enjoyment food? Let's say that you're going to a restaurant for dinner. What do they typically offer before the server takes your order? Usually bread (with butter) or tortilla chips (with salsas). If you decide to use your enjoyment food for this meal, wait until you've eaten your vegetables and proteins before you eat the bread or tortilla chips. Your eyes may be hungrier than your stomach, so you might end up eating all of the bread servings (along with the butter) even before your drinks come out.

A new study published in *Diabetes Care* finds that eating bread after your meal can blunt the rise in blood sugar and reduce the appetite. In the study, Louis Aronne and his colleagues served participants a meal of grilled chicken, steam vegetables, and a salad dressed with vinaigrette. First, participants ate a standard-sized ciabatta roll. Then, the participants ate the same meal, except the bread was served last. On average, the participants' peak blood glucose and one hour postprandial (after meal) insulin levels were 29 percent and 50 percent lower respectively when they ate the bread after their meal.

It's even worse if you have refined carbohydrates on an empty stomach because there's nothing to slow down the breakdown of that carbohydrate into sugar, resulting in a spike in blood glucose and an increase in appetite.

Therefore, the best time to have your enjoyment food is after you finish your vegetables and proteins. By filling up with grilled salmon and steamed asparagus, you're far less likely to overeat the bread. To go back to the earlier example, ask them to bring back the oven-warmed bread later on *after* you've finished your meal. Even then, consider choosing wheat over white bread.

Similarly, if you want pizza during the Passive Phase, you may have one slice of pizza. Make sure to eat your vegetables and proteins first before you reach for that piece.

A common mistake you might make is to reduce the vegetables and protein portion from the Active to the Passive Phase. You might believe that if you're eating grains, you're packing more calories, so you need to reduce your protein intake. That's the old way of thinking in terms of calories alone. If you think in terms of insulin, you understand the point of keeping the same amount of vegetable and protein intake during the Passive Phase so that you can minimize the insulin spike. If you feel satisfied, you're less likely to overindulge on the grains, starchy vegetables, high-GI fruits, or sweets.

SAMANTHA'S STORY

We've covered a lot of material up to this point. Let's put these concepts into clinical practice.

Samantha, a fifty-two-year-old government worker, didn't cheat during the four months of the Active Phase. She lost 33 pounds, or about 14 percent of her body weight. She hit the weight-loss plateau, but she still wanted to lose another 20 pounds. When we introduced the concept of raising her insulin level to help her overcome this plateau, she was very hesitant and nervous.

"I don't miss eating rice anymore," she shared. "I want to stick to what I'm eating now." She explained further that she had worked so hard to get to this point that she didn't want to risk gaining back her weight. We went over the rationale for increasing the insulin level again during the Passive Phase, as she had already reached her plateau. We showed her weight the past few visits to be constant as further proof that she wouldn't be able to lose additional weight by staying the same course. We reassured her that as long as she stuck to the regimen, her weight gain would be minimal, if at all. But she must slowly introduce back her enjoyment food for the next few weeks.

Samantha started the first two weeks by eating half a cup of oatmeal for breakfast. On other days, she would eat a slice of bread while still eating a salad and plenty of meat on her sandwich. On some nights, she would enjoy half a scoop of rice along with her salmon and grilled asparagus.

Two weeks into the Passive Phase, she came back to weigh in, and the scale showed she had lost another pound. For the next two weeks, Samantha ate a portion of enjoyment food per day at breakfast, lunch, or dinner. She shared that she had lobster ravioli at a local restaurant one day. It had been months since she had eaten it. Because she knew she wanted to order that, her favorite dish, she ate two hard-boiled egg whites for breakfast, a handful of grapes for a morning snack, a salad with grilled chicken breast for lunch, and a handful of almonds for her afternoon snack. Before she ordered dinner, the waiter brought out some bread with a delicious spread. At first, Samantha reached for the bread, but decided that she didn't want to waste her enjoyment food on bread. She really wanted the lobster ravioli. So she asked that her salad be brought out as soon as possible. Instead of getting fries, she asked the waiter to replace them with steamed vegetables to go along with her lobster ravioli.

After four weeks, she came back to the office for a weigh-in. She noticed that she had gained a pound since her last visit. We reviewed her food choices. She had continued to drink water or unsweetened iced tea and stuck to fruits and nuts for her snacks. She ate only one portion of enjoyment food per day. While she was disappointed that she had actually gained weight, we reminded her that her goal in the Passive Phase had switched to maintaining her weight. We went over how much more enjoyment food she could have the next two weeks, up to one and a half portions per day. She was still a bit nervous but determined to stay on track. She was very conscientious to keep the amount of her vegetable and protein intake the same. She came back two weeks later and was happy to see that her weight remained unchanged.

Samantha shared that her birthday was coming up in a week and she wanted to eat some birthday cake. She would be able to eat a slice of her favorite cake that day but no other carbs, even though she was up to one portion of carbs for the next two weeks.

Now that Samantha was six weeks into the Passive Phase, she was able to eat up to two portions of enjoyment food per day. She was happy that this time period corresponded to her upcoming birthday, so she was able to reintroduce sweets into her meals. Typically, she would eat a cup of oatmeal sprinkled with fresh berries for breakfast. Depending on her schedule, she would typically eat brown rice or whole-grain bread either for lunch or dinner. She would forgo eating hamburger buns and stick to consuming a lettuce-wrapped protein burger before she ate the fries. But on her birthday, she really wanted to eat a slice of chocolate cake. So that day, she made sure that her breakfast and lunch consisted only of foods that didn't spike her insulin level. She knew that a sweet is equivalent to two portions of enjoyment food, so she only ordered a filet steak with grilled asparagus for dinner. She was ready for that slice of chocolate cake. She ate it without feeling any guilt since she followed through on her game plan perfectly. Sure enough, when Samantha came back to weigh in at week eight, the scale remained relatively stable.

She continued to have two portions of enjoyment food per day for her third month of the Passive Phase. When she wanted sweets, she would plan her day ahead of time, making sure that the sweets were the only enjoyment food she had for that day. After three months of slowly raising her insulin level, she gained two pounds since she first reintroduced her enjoyment food. This is reasonable given that she was eating grains, starchy vegetables, and sweets again.

It could've been a lot worse if she didn't follow through with this game plan.

What about exercise? Certainly, had Samantha exercised more to burn off the extra calories from the grains, starchy vegetables, or sweets, she might not have gained weight at all. Even though the increase in insulin level tells your body to store fat, if you're able to neutralize the increased intake of calories from the extra enjoyment food with exercise, your body doesn't store fat simply because there are no extra calories to store as fat. We'll talk more in detail in the next chapter on the importance of exercise in the Passive Phase.

Samantha is now ready to go back to the Active Phase again. She still wants to lose another twenty pounds. Because her insulin level is higher now than when she ended the first Active Phase, her body will start to burn fat again as she drops her insulin level. Let's say if Samantha is happy with her weight and she would like to maintain it, she would just continue the Passive Phase by eating two portions of enjoyment food per day and exercising three times per week.

As you can see from this case, it's important to plan your day when you're going through the Passive Phase. You need to be aware of where you're at so that you know exactly how much enjoyment food you're able to add back to your daily life. We highly recommend you weigh yourself weekly. Always try to pick the same day to weigh in. This way, it will remind you that you can increase your portion of enjoyment food. In addition, the regular weigh-in will help you keep track of your weight.

What happens if you deviate from the game plan and gain too much weight? How much weight gain is too much? A simple rule to remember here is five pounds. If at any point during the Passive Phase you gain five pounds or more, you must go back to the Active Phase and drop your insulin level until your weight gain stabilizes. Then, go back to the Passive Phase by adding back half a portion of enjoyment food and work your way back up from the beginning, and go for three months.

It *is* possible to eat sweets without regaining weight. If you're only introducing a portion of grains, starchy vegetables, or sweets after you're full from eating vegetables and proteins, you'll be able to minimize your weight gain. And if you're limiting the sweets to only once a day, rather than allowing yourself to eat them anytime you want, it also minimizes the potential for weight gain. You see, it's quite simple! It makes sense and it's very effective.

Chapter 12

EXERCISE IN THE PASSIVE PHASE

Once you hit the weight-loss plateau and enter the Passive Phase, exercise becomes more critical. According to data from the National Weight Control Registry, people who had lost at least 10 percent of their body weight and kept it off for one year reported high levels of physical activity as part of their weight-loss strategy. Continued adherence to exercise was a key strategy for long-term success in keeping off the weight.

You have to exercise more in the Passive than in the Active Phase to minimize the weight regain—thirty minutes a day, three times per week. When you're gently increasing your insulin level by strategically reintroducing grains, starchy vegetables, and high-GI fruits, you have to exercise more to burn off extra calories in order to prevent weight gain. If you don't burn off the extra calories, they'll be converted to fat due to the elevated insulin level. On the other hand, if you burn off the extra calories, there won't be any calories left to convert to fat. In simple terms, the more you exercise, the less likely it is that you'll regain your weight.

You might wonder why we're discussing calories. It's true, from the beginning, we said that with Thinsulin, you don't think in terms of calories, but in terms of insulin. Is what we're teaching you now contradicting that? The answer is no!

Remember, your goals are different depending on what phase you're in. In the Active Phase, you're lowering your insulin level; in the Passive Phase, you'll be increasing your insulin level. You'll always need to think in terms of insulin in both phases. In the Passive Phase, you're choosing only one enjoyment food at breakfast, lunch, or dinner to allow your insulin level to spike. That enjoyment food is on top of what you've been eating during the Active Phase. Therefore, your total caloric intake is going to be higher. You need to take these extra calories into account. The best way to neutralize these extra calories is through exercise. You see, it's not that we don't believe in calories. Ultimately, reducing your calories will lead to weight loss. We're just asking you not to think in terms of calories. When you choose proteins and green, leafy vegetables, guess what? These foods are much lower in calories than bread, pasta, or potatoes. So when you think in terms of insulin, you'll automatically select foods that are low in calories.

WHAT KIND OF EXERCISE SHOULD I DO?

You can do any kind you like. Of course, make sure you enjoy your physical activity. If you don't like running on a treadmill, go jogging outside. If you don't like running, you might choose to do kickboxing, dance classes, or yoga. Just make sure it's at least thirty minutes per day, three times per week.

Whatever you do, don't make time an excuse *not* to exercise. If something comes up and you get off-schedule, don't use that as an excuse to scrap your workouts for the week. Don't fall into the all-or-nothing thinking. Instead, choose to do other physical activities even for the limited time that you're able to.

WHEN TO EXERCISE

When is the best time of day to exercise? There's a difference in opinion. A study at Appalachian State University reported that participants who exercised in the morning slept better at night and reduced their blood pressure throughout the day. Dr. S. R. Collier and his research assistants compared individuals ages forty to sixty exercising moderately for thirty minutes, three times a week, at either 7 a.m., 1 p.m., or 7 p.m. The participants who exercised in the morning had deeper sleep cycles, spending up to 75 percent more time in the reparative sleep stage, than those who exercised at other times in the day.

Another study found that people who exercised in the afternoon performed better. The researchers analyzed a group of cyclists who worked out at 6 a.m. or 6 p.m. They found that the group that exercised in the evening boosted workout performance.

It's important to consider the timing of your exercise and when you're eating. It makes sense not to do strenuous exercise after you eat a full meal at lunch or dinner. You might remember your parents telling you as kids not to swim or run after eating lunch or dinner. Instead, take a leisurely stroll after lunch or dinner for thirty minutes.

It's best to do strenuous exercise in a fasted state. Research has shown that your body burns a greater percentage of fat for fuel during exercise on an empty stomach. If you ate, the body would rely on the carbohydrates from food for fuel so it wouldn't burn that much fat. Based on this research study, probably the only time you're in a fasted state is early in the morning before breakfast.

You might be worried that you'll feel weak if you haven't eaten anything prior to a long bike ride in the morning. If so, consider eating protein such as egg whites or chicken and green, leafy vegetables. Even though you're not in a fasted state, at least what you're eating won't spike your insulin level. This still forces your body to burn body fat. The harder you work out, the more proteins such as lean meat you should eat prior to the workout. Don't grab that protein bar. It might be low in sugar and high in protein, but it's not as good as eating lean chicken breast or green veggies.

In short, if you have the discipline to wake up early to run, swim, or bike, that's great! Not only will this help your body burn fat, but it will also help to improve your sleep at night. In addition, it sets the right tone for the day as you feel like you have a higher energy level. If you can't wake up early to exercise, don't worry. Just exercise at whatever time you find most convenient for you. Once you develop a new exercise routine, it'll get easier for you to develop a new habit. Practice makes a better you.

THINSULIN
PASSIVE PHASE MILESTONES

In this phase, you'll increase your insulin level while maintaining your weight. The first purpose is to help you overcome the weight-loss plateau. After three months, you can go back to the Active Phase and lower your insulin level. The second purpose of the Passive Phase is to help you maintain your weight. If you're happy with your weight, you can continue with the Passive Phase to keep your weight off.

WEEKS 17–20

"I eat for enjoyment." You should hit the weight-loss plateau by the end of four months on the Active Phase. Before you can reintroduce grains, starchy vegetables, or high-GI fruits to increase your insulin level, you need to change your thinking from "I enjoy eating" to "I eat for enjoyment." You need to enjoy your food, but you can only have your enjoyment food after you finish your green, leafy vegetables, and proteins at breakfast, lunch, or dinner.

Reintroduce grains, starchy vegetables, or high-GI fruits.

1. Continue to eat five times per day.
   - Breakfast: 1 portion of dairy product (only at breakfast), protein meat or seafood, or egg white
   - Morning snack: 1 portion of fresh, low-GI fruit (apple, orange, grapes, or berries)

- Lunch: At least 1 portion of green, leafy vegetables and at least 1 portion of protein meat or seafood
- Afternoon snack: 1 portion of raw nuts
- Dinner: At least 1 portion of green, leafy vegetables and at least 1 portion of protein meat or seafood

2. You may add half a portion of enjoyment food for the day to breakfast, lunch, or dinner for the first two weeks of the Passive Phase (Weeks 17–18). The enjoyment food can be grains, high-GI fruits (an extra fruit or any fruits besides apple, orange, grapes, or berries), or starchy vegetables (potatoes, corn, carrots, or beets). You may increase to one portion of enjoyment food for the day during Weeks 19–20.

3. Don't add any sweets back to your regimen at this time.

4. Increase your physical activity. By this time, you need to do your aerobic exercise for at least thirty minutes three times a week.

5. Make sure to weigh yourself once every week. If you've gained more than 5 pounds since you started the Passive Phase, you need to go back to the Active Phase for one month.

WEEKS 21–24

Start with one and a half portions per day for Weeks 21–22 before you increase to two total portions of enjoyment food per day (Week 23–24).

1. If you're staying on track and maintaining your weight, you can now add two total portions of enjoyment food per day.

2. The two portions of enjoyment food cannot be eaten at the same meal.

3. Make sure you're eating green, leafy vegetables first, proteins second, and then enjoyment food last. By eating vegetables and proteins first, you're less likely to overeat the enjoyment food.

WEEKS 25–28

Continue two portions of enjoyment food per day. Remember that sweets are equivalent to two portions per day of grains, starchy vegetables, or high-GI fruits. Sweets are *not* to be used in addition to the portions above.

1. Continue to weigh yourself. If you've gained more than 5 pounds since you started the Passive Phase, you need to go back to the Active Phase for one month.
2. If you're staying on track, be prepared to make a decision. By week 28, or about seven months after you've started the Thinsulin Program, your body has hit the set point where you'll be able to lose weight again.

WEEK 29

1. If you want to lose more weight and burn fat, you can go back to the Active Phase.
2. If you're happy with your weight, just continue along the Passive Phase and eat no more than two portions of enjoyment food. Make sure to weigh yourself weekly to see how many pounds you've gained since you've started the Passive Phase.

PART V
STICKING WITH IT AND STAYING THIN FOR LIFE

Chapter 13

STAYING ON TRACK

Success on Thinsulin, like any other treatment, requires two things: an understanding of the concepts and the internal motivation to make changes in your life.

Physicians typically measure the likelihood of success in following a treatment plan in terms of compliance or adherence. These terms are often used interchangeably, but there's a difference. *Compliance* implies that an individual, often with little understanding, abides by the advice of a health care provider without question. *Adherence* involves the collaboration between the individual and health care provider to achieve a goal such as weight loss. A person adherent to treatment follows an agreed upon therapeutic treatment, rather than blindly following the advice (compliance). People adherent to treatment are more likely to be successful with it.

When you first start a weight-loss program, you're at greatest risk for non-adherence. Unless you start to see some results, you're less likely to continue the regimen. In fact, adherence to a weight-loss program is correlated with the degree of weight loss. The more weight you lose, the more likely you're going to adhere to the regimen. But that can change rather quickly if you become complacent and allow your bad habits and old ways of thinking back into your life. Long-term adherence is determined by knowledge and motivation.

Knowledge includes health literacy, which is defined as "the ability to read, understand, and act on health information." You're less likely to follow a program if you have a tough time understanding the instructions. If you learn more about the science and concepts behind the program, along with the techniques, you're more likely to stay on track. Research studies show that knowledge and health literacy are associated with compliance rates. This is why we spent a lot of time explaining the scientific principles behind the Thinsulin Program in this book.

Research has also shown that motivation plays a key role in the success of weight loss and maintenance. The combination of a willingness to change along with a social support network determines motivation. If you're not willing to change, you'll have a thousand reasons why you can't start. You're simply not ready—and that's OK. A time will come in your life when you'll know you're ready. Changes often come slowly, often in small steps. Sometimes, you may need to fail several times before you're truly committed to change. During that time, a strong social support network can make it easier for you to get back on your feet and stay motivated.

WHAT'S YOUR ADHERENCE LEVEL?

Where do you stand right now? You can assess yourself quickly. We adapted the principles from the Case Management Adherence Guidelines published in June 2006 to create the Adherence Intention Quadrant to predict adherence rate. In this Adherence Intention box, each quadrant assesses the level of motivation and knowledge as high or low to see how likely you're going to stay on track. The goal is to get to Quadrant 1, where you have both high motivation and knowledge. Quadrant 1 predicts the highest rate of adherence while Quadrant 4 (low motivation and knowledge) predicts the lowest rate of adherence. The other two quadrants lack either knowledge or motivation, which puts you at risk for non-adherence.

Let's take Quadrant 2 as an example. Perhaps you're highly motivated to make changes, but low knowledge is your downfall. You

ADHERENCE INTENTION	

Q1   **High** Motivation
       High Knowledge
	Q2 **High** Motivation
	       Low Knowledge

Q3   **Low** Motivation
       High Knowledge
	Q4 **Low** Motivation
	       Low Knowledge

may be motivated to start a new juicing diet, but you're not likely to encounter success if you add carrots and beets to your kale, spinach, and celery. A lack of knowledge about the effect of beets and carrots on insulin will leave you pondering why you can't seem to lose weight even though you're drinking a very "healthy" juice daily. Like a domino effect, your motivation decreases when you're seeing minimal results with juicing.

On the other hand, you might have high knowledge in Quadrant 3, but your motivation is low. You might know all the foods that spike insulin, but if you're not ready to change, that knowledge doesn't necessarily translate to action. You need both motivation and knowledge for you to adhere to treatment.

Your weight-loss journey will have many ups and downs. It may take you through many turns, depending on what life throws at you. So you need to be ready by knowing where you're at in the adherence quadrant. If you don't understand or if you forget a concept, make sure you go back to read that chapter again. You don't want to continue blindly without knowing why you're doing something. Figure out where the misunderstanding occurs and correct it.

BOOSTING YOUR KNOWLEDGE

The concepts of Thinsulin are easy to grasp, but it takes time to master the technique to break down the foods into the five groups. If you don't do it correctly, you won't be able to lower your insulin level and you'll be stuck at that weight for a while.

For example, a common mistake you might make is to assume that all salads are healthy. Salad can be healthy, but it depends what's in it. You can't simply say it's a salad and it belongs to the vegetable group. You still need to break down the contents in the salad and put them in the five groups. You would group the croutons into the grains group, dried cranberries into the fruit group, and lettuce, shredded carrots, and beets into the vegetable group. After you group them, you see if the foods increase insulin level or not. You remember that only a handful of *fresh* berries won't spike your insulin level. That eliminates the dried cranberries (which are often sweetened with sugar as well). The same can be said for the croutons. Even healthy grains will still spike your insulin level. As for the salad, the romaine lettuce and spinach won't spike your insulin level, but the carrots and beets will.

You need to do the same for any new dishes that you want to try. Don't just look at the meat or seafood dish and assume that it's OK to eat. Find out how they marinate the fish and how they cook it. For example, if you're looking at the menu and you have a choice between a salmon or sea bass dish, read the description a bit more and try to break it down further. The teriyaki salmon contains brown sugar and it may spike your insulin level, while the steamed sea bass marinated with soy sauce may not spike your insulin level. It's easy to overlook these details.

One helpful technique is to record what you're eating in a food log, either by using web-based apps or keeping a food diary. However you choose to keep records, that's OK. You just have to do it so that you're forced to slow down and group the foods. Some of our patients in our clinics prefer to take pictures of their meals using their smartphones. A picture is worth a thousand words. Our patients email us the pictures and we tell them if they're doing it correctly. This is such a simple yet effective technique to help them make adjustments quickly. You may apply this technique and share your photos on the Thinsulin Facebook page. Other Thinsulin readers may give you feedback on lowering your insulin correctly.

Another effective technique is to be a teacher. You only truly know a subject when you're able to teach it. You may think you know it, but if you're unable to explain the Thinsulin concepts to your family or friends, you have yet to master the knowledge.

We want you to put in your own words a short summary of Thinsulin that you can use to teach others. Emphasize in this summary that Thinsulin isn't a diet. It's a program that teaches them to think in terms of insulin. What happens if you cheat? Show them how you're breaking down the foods you're eating into five groups and figuring out what spikes your insulin level. If you don't remember this, go back to the earlier chapters and reread them so that you truly know these concepts. By teaching others, your knowledge increases, allowing you to better apply these concepts to your daily life.

Motivation is a bit more challenging to address. It's not as easy as reading some materials to increase knowledge. Hopefully, some of the stories here inspire you to change, but it requires more than just stories to sustain that motivation over time or even to get started. The use of motivational interviewing (MI) can help inspire you to begin, while having a strong social support network will help you to stay on course.

MI is taught to clinicians to help their patients. So the purpose of sharing these principles with you isn't so much teaching you how to do your own therapy as it is allowing you a glimpse through the eyes of a psychiatrist to see how this process works. Many therapists out there are trained at MI. Ask your insurance providers for a list of therapists in your area if you'd like to pursue MI therapy.

MOTIVATIONAL INTERVIEWING

MI is a style of counseling used by clinicians to help identify and engage your intrinsic motivation for change. Rather than telling you what to do, the method uses nonjudgmental and nonconfrontational techniques to help you take the first step toward change. MI has been shown to increase motivation and adherence to medication regimen for many illnesses. When applied to weight management, the goal of MI isn't just limited to weight loss, but also to understanding the process that leads to change. MI utilizes four key steps to increase motivation:

Engage. Rather than telling you what to do, it's important for the clinicians to ask open-ended questions, express empathy, and listen to your concerns.

Focus. After you share your concerns, a clinician keeps you focused to identify a behavior to change.

Evoke a response. A clinician discusses with you any perceived barriers to change while addressing your ambivalence and readiness to change.

Plan. The last step is to help develop a realistic plan for you to start.

An important influence on motivation is affirmation of being heard. *Empathy* plays a key role in this process. Many times, the words *sympathy* and *empathy* are used synonymously incorrectly. We'll tell you an example to illustrate the difference. Randy shared in a group session about John, his younger brother, who struggles with schizophrenia. It was very touching as Randy described how John was forced to drop out of school at the age of twenty-two, became homeless, and tried to kill himself, all because John suffers from delusions and hallucinations associated with his illness.

Randy, a thirty-two-year-old small business owner, told a group of other parents and patients with schizophrenia in the group, "I don't want any sympathy for my brother." Everyone in the group was a bit shocked by that statement, given the fact that they'd just listened to John's difficulty in life.

"I want people to have empathy for my brother," Randy continued. He further explained, "I don't want you to feel sorry for my brother. I want you to put yourself in his shoes. When you pity him, you have essentially written him off and given him very little chance to succeed. But when you have empathy and put yourself in his shoes to see his struggles, you'll give him more hope to succeed in life."

When it comes to treating obesity, we need to do the same and put ourselves in the shoes of obese and overweight individuals. In our practices, patients tell us so often of their struggles with obesity. Even though they may have been successful in many aspects of their life, their inability to control their weight represents an *unspoken failure* in their life. No matter how successful they are as businesswomen, housewives, students, or firemen, they literally carry this failure everywhere they go. Everyone around them sees it, too, with every pound that they gain. They feel embarrassment and shame. The multiple failures with different diets further reinforces this self-perception.

Let's apply the MI steps to help someone you know who's struggling to lose weight because they don't have the motivation to start Thinsulin. Let's call this person Mary.

Engage: First, show empathy. Acknowledge to Mary that it's hard to lose weight. Let Mary know she is not alone. Millions of Americans out there have the same struggle. Next, don't tell Mary to lose weight. Instead, ask her what benefits she may have if she loses ten pounds? How would she feel to actually achieve that weight-loss goal? What's holding her back? Acknowledge that there are many reasons why she's unable to start a program right now. Maybe she's too busy with work, school, or family. Maybe the holidays or a birthday are coming up. All perfectly rational reasons.

Focus: After you hear Mary's concerns, help her focus by identifying a behavior to change. Start with giving up sweets as drinks. Ask for a one-week commitment. Yes, only one week. Not forever! Not a month. Just one week. Thinking of it as a short time frame can be much more doable than all-or-nothing thinking such as, "I can't *ever* have sweets, period."

Evoke a response: You can address Mary's ambivalence and readiness to change. What are the barriers to prevent this change? Oftentimes, the barriers aren't actually real, but more so perceived to be real. For example, Mary can easily misinterpret this to think that she can't have sweets for the rest of her life. That's her fear, but simply not the reality. If you sense resistance to even a week of commitment, then ask Mary to give up sodas for a day. Yes, one single day. You want her to get started. If she makes that commitment, at least she has a chance to succeed. If she doesn't start, there is zero chance of success.

Plan: Develop a realistic plan for Mary to start. Tell her to get rid of all soda from her home, work, and vehicle. Next, encourage her to fill up a big water bottle with water. Minimize any excuses that she may come up with to drink soda. Even put that water bottle in the car the night before so that she can't say that she didn't have any water the next day.

As you can see from the example above of how MI works, it's worthwhile to reemphasize the importance of empathy. If someone you care about is obese, remember to listen closely to what they're saying and *affirm* this struggle. Don't make a value judgment. Instead, elicit their reactions by inquiring, "Could you do this?" or "Does this make sense?" Don't tell them what to do. It might be better to ask them to be partners in their journey. In addition, using self-motivating statements such as "You can do it," "You've done it before," and "Keep up the good work" can help boost their confidence to stay on track. Having strong social support will also help to sustain their motivation.

It may be helpful for you to apply some of the MI principles in your life. When you feel unmotivated, don't be too harsh on yourself. Search for any recent changes in your life that may have led you to overeat and gain weight. Rather than beating yourself up, have empathy for yourself and try to focus on changing that behavior. Figure out the barriers that prevent you from changing and develop a realistic plan for you to start.

Some commercial weight-loss programs use weekly follow-up visits to provide social support and hold people accountable. Indeed, it is important to have personal accountability, such as weighing yourself regularly.

Your weekly weigh-in can be anywhere, not just at a doctor's office or in a weight-loss program. The idea is to set away time from your busy schedule to reflect on your journey.

Doing a weekly weigh-in can be valuable beyond just holding you accountable. If you use that time for *self-reflection* on your journey, this may help you sustain your motivation over time. The weekly visit forces you to take time away from your busy schedule so that you can focus on *yourself* rather than your work and family. When you make time to weigh in, you're saying to yourself and others that your health is just as important as all your other life commitments. It offers the time to think of your goals and measure your commitment to your health. If you have reasons (excuses) that put your job or friends above your health, remind yourself that without good health, you won't be able to help anyone. Think of what you hear before you depart on a plane: "In case of a sudden drop in air cabin pressure, make sure you put on the oxygen mask *first* before you help others."

SOCIAL SUPPORT

A research study conducted at the University of Illinois reported that being accountable to other people was critical in their success. Having a good social support network can help boost your motivation. The help and encouragement provided by your family, friends, or coworkers defines social support. So share this concept with your social support as this may motivate you even more to stay on track. Encourage your friend or partner to do Thinsulin with you as it's less daunting than doing it by yourself.

While social support can help motivate you to start, social support has shown to be very effective in keeping the weight off by enhancing feelings of confidence and control.

Each weight-loss program may appeal to some and not to others. It really depends on you. Whatever program you choose, it's important to enlist friends and families as part of your support system. A study showed that when participants enrolled with their friends in a weight-loss program, they were more likely to keep off the weight compared with those who attended one on their own.

On the flip side, the lack of support can harm your goals. For example, your friends or family members may respond negatively, sabotaging any progress that you make. Or, if your support system doesn't understand your program, it would be difficult not to cheat if they continue to bring ice cream and sodas to you. So be sure that your family and friends understand the Thinsulin guidelines and will be supportive of you in your weight-loss efforts.

MENTORSHIP

During the Thinsulin Passive Phase, at this stage, you already have a strong foundation of knowledge about insulin and weight loss. You may also begin teaching these concepts to others. Your last task is to select a mentee who wants to learn from you. Teach that mentee everything that you know and guide the mentee through any treacherous pitfalls.

The idea behind mentorship is to truly hold you accountable to yourself and others. The fact that your mentee looks up to you for advice and encouragement will only help you to stay on course so that you can serve as their role model. When you're slipping, a mentee's innocent questions may pull you back onto the right path. As a mentor, you'll find joy when you see how confident your mentee feels after losing all that weight. This will motivate you to continue to set a good example because you simply won't want to disappoint them.

As you embark on this journey, you won't be traveling alone. Along the way, you will learn a lot, but you'll also have the opportunity to teach as well. Once you've mastered the concepts, you'll mentor others to help them learn and implement the Thinsulin Program.

Chapter 14

BREAKING BAD HABITS

"Motivation is what gets you started. Habit is what keeps you going."

—JIM RYUN

Imagine if you couldn't form habits. You would have to motivate yourself anew every single time you wanted to exercise or choose insulin-safe foods. Getting started is always the hardest part of any new regimen. But the good news is, you can create new habits that over time make following the Thinsulin Program easy.

Habits can arise through repetition and are a normal part of life. They're developed when good or enjoyable events trigger the brain's reward systems involving a neurotransmitter or brain chemical called dopamine. Habit affects how you start your morning, what you eat, and how you approach your work. You might notice that some baseball players have elaborate routines that they often perform before they bat.

Habits can be good or bad. A good habit doesn't cause any harmful effects in your life. A bad habit can result in harmful addictions or even multiple addictions such as smoking, alcohol, and/or drug abuse, gambling, and/or overeating.

According to Charles Duhigg, author of *The Power of Habit: Why We Do What We Do In Life and Business*, at the core of every habit is a neurological loop located in the basal ganglia of the brain. It's also known as a "habit loop," and consists of three parts—cue, routine, and reward. The cue, or trigger, initiates the routine, which is rewarded to continue the habit loop. Habits become routine so that your brain can devote attention to something else without you being mentally aware of it. For example, you can brush your teeth while reading a book.

Habits are modified in a similar way. A new trigger might alter the routine, which is rewarded to reinforce the habit. For example, a woman might change her eating habits due to cravings during pregnancy. Prior to pregnancy, Quincy, a twenty-eight-year-old dentist, had very healthy eating habits. She didn't drink sodas or eat sweets. Early during her second pregnancy, however, she developed cravings for sweets. Besides eating regular meals, she would go on ice cream binges and craved candy throughout her pregnancy. The sugar cravings stopped after she delivered her baby, but her poor eating habits did not. She was used to eating a certain way and found it difficult to get back to her previous, healthier eating habits.

Bad habits might be hard to change, but it can be done. It's simply a matter of understanding how habits are formed and modified. You can change habits by addressing the "habit loop." You need to identify the trigger, change your routine, and find a way to reward this new routine. This might sound simple enough, but they're just words. How do you convert words into actions? You can use behavioral therapy, also known as *behavioral modification*, to help break bad habits and form new ones.

Behavioral therapy works by changing the behaviors that aren't serving you well, known as *maladaptive behaviors*. Because maladaptive behaviors are learned, you can "unlearn" them and replace them with new behaviors. It's based on principles of learning: classical conditioning and operant conditioning.

Classical conditioning says that eating is triggered by events in life (cues) that are strongly linked to food intake. Therefore, if you can identify your cues that trigger eating and learn new responses to them, you can change your eating habits.

Operant conditioning, developed by psychologist Dr. B. F. Skinner, is guided by the principle that behaviors are shaped by positive reinforcement or negative, punishing stimuli. Positive reinforcement through reward encourages certain behaviors, while negative reinforcement through punishment discourages undesirable behaviors. (A classic example, you might recall from a psychology 101 class, is when a rat receives an electric shock as a punishment.)

Behavioral therapy has been shown to be effective in weight loss. A review of fifty-eight clinical trials using behavioral therapy as part of the weight-loss program showed more weight loss (7 pounds) than the groups that didn't receive behavioral therapy over a twelve-to-eighteen-month period. Structured approaches such as food plans, meal replacements, or pharmacotherapy have been shown to help increase the magnitude of the weight loss somewhat, but not by much (less than 3 to 5 kilograms or 6.6 to 11 pounds difference after twelve to eighteen months of treatment).

But given today's fast-paced environment that encourages over-consumption of high-calorie foods, it's difficult to overcome these barriers and adopt a new set of skills using behavioral therapy alone. In addition, we also know that factors other than behavior, such as genetics, psychology, and metabolism, affect obesity. This is why Thinsulin's combination approach—the biopsychosocial approach to weight management—makes the most sense. To be successful, it's important to address the biological, psychological, and behavioral issues together as a whole, rather than as separate issues. This will help you develop a set of skills to achieve weight loss or to maintain your weight.

In this chapter, you'll learn how the Thinsulin Program uses the principles of behavioral therapy to go along with the biology of insulin and the psychology of CBT to change your thinking. You can learn to adjust to the program's new way of eating through the process of goal setting, self-monitoring, feedback, and reinforcement.

GOAL SETTING

When you decide to lose weight, you want to lose as many pounds as you possibly can. Many times, your expectations don't match the realities of obtainable results. Losing 10 percent of your weight is considered a success, as you significantly reduce the risk of medical problems such as high blood pressure and diabetes. However, many people aren't happy with a 10-percent weight loss. Rather, they seek weight losses of approximately 30 percent reduction in their body weight. That's simply unrealistic in such a short amount of time.

In the Active Phase, you can expect to lose at least three to five pounds in the first week. On average, you'll end up losing between 10 to 15 percent of your body weight after four months before you hit the weight-loss plateau. If you stay on track, you might lose about 20 percent of your body weight after four months. That would be awesome, but the focus shouldn't be on how much weight you lose weekly. It's more important that you set simple goals one week at a time. Focus on eating five times a day. Make sure you eat breakfast, snack or a fruit, have lunch, snack or nuts, and eat dinner. If you continue this eating pattern for four months, this will become your new eating habit.

In addition, focus on thinking in terms of insulin. With each meal, make sure you categorize the foods into five groups. Then, choose the foods that won't spike your insulin level. Do this daily for every meal and you'll see the weight loss. Every week that you lose weight will serve as positive reinforcement. If you cheat even just once to spike your insulin level, you won't lose weight despite working hard the entire week to stay on track. This serves as negative reinforcement, with the punishment a static weight scale.

Don't get frustrated if you're not losing as much weight as you expect. You'll lose the most weight within the first month and lose less weight in the ensuing months. If you're not seeing any weight loss for two weeks, write down what you're eating. Analyze the food as if you're a chef making it so that you know which ingredients are added.

Brad, a twenty-four-year-old student, was losing weight steadily on the Active Phase for the first two months. His weight then stabilized for two weeks. His eating log showed that he'd been eating Korean barbequed beef twice a week. Brad didn't understand why he wasn't losing weight because he was just eating beef—which is protein, right? When he Googled "how to marinate Korean barbequed beef," he realized that 2.5 pounds of rib-eye beef contains at least two tablespoons of brown sugar and one tablespoon of rice wine. This explains why cooking the beef on the grill leaves a brownish residue. The brown sugar and rice wine sure spiked his insulin level, leaving him stuck at that weight. Brad continued to go to the Korean restaurant, but he stopped ordering the marinated beef and ate only the unmarinated meat. Soon after, he was able to lose weight again.

Once you hit the weight-loss plateau, your goal in the Passive Phase shifts to slowly increasing your insulin level while maintaining your weight. It's important to remember this or you're going to be disappointed if you don't lose weight. That's not your goal during this phase! Yes, you need to add one portion of enjoyment food to increase your insulin level. Still, focus on thinking in terms of insulin so that you'll have one enjoyment food after you have your vegetables and proteins at breakfast, lunch, or dinner. A normal tendency is to cut down on proteins during the Passive Phase. Make sure you still have at least one portion of proteins.

Don't look too far ahead. Set your goals one week at a time. If you're able to stick to this plan and maintain about the same weight at the end of the week, you're doing a terrific job. If you gain a pound or two, assess how much enjoyment food you're having and when you're having it. Consider increasing your physical activity. If at any time you gain more than five pounds since you started the Passive Phase, don't panic! Whatever you do, don't fall into the trap of all-or-nothing thinking. Most likely, you're deviating from the plan by having more enjoyment food or eating it as a snack. Go back to the Active Phase for three weeks to drop your insulin level again. You'll see your weight gain stabilize and oftentimes, you'll be able to lose the five pounds that you recently gained. After you're back on track, go back to the Passive Phase, but this time around, try your best to follow the program.

SELF-MONITORING

Self-monitoring is a component of behavioral therapy that has been proven to be effective in achieving better weight control. The goal of self-monitoring is to increase self-awareness of your behavior through observation and the recording of your eating and exercise patterns. When you self-monitor, you begin to pay attention to triggers, notice barriers, and identify challenges to changing your behavior. It serves as an early warning system to help you correct your course rather than beat yourself up for not attaining a goal. Self-monitoring can help you to identify positive behaviors that will keep you on track rather than relying on negative self-judgment to stay motivated.

Commonly used self-monitoring techniques include keeping food logs or diaries, or weighing oneself regularly. Record what you eat and drink daily, including the type, amount, and calories. You can either document in a journal or use online programs to help you track the foods as well as calories. These online websites are easy to use and can tell you exactly how much you're eating a day.

A food diary is more detailed than a food log because it might contain your stress level, moods, or feelings surrounding eating or triggers for eating. Recognizing the triggers or emotions associated with eating can provide real-life feedback to help you change. If you're a stress eater who turns to ice cream, having a food diary can help you to recognize this pattern, so that you know to rid your freezer of ice cream during, say, tax time, midterm exams, or other stressful events. Some technologically advanced individuals might blog their food diary online to keep track of their progress.

Food logs and diaries are only helpful for the long-term, however, if they are used regularly. If you're the type of person who likes keeping logs or diaries, go for it. But don't just do it for the sake of doing it. Make sure you take the time to review your food logs or diaries and figure out why, when, and how you got off track. Once you gain the self-awareness, you might find new ways to change that behavior.

If you're *not* the type of person to keep logs or diaries, don't worry. The Thinsulin Program also incorporates self-monitoring techniques to help you. Instead of logging the food types and calories, you need to monitor your hunger level and cravings. If you crave desserts after dinner, then you know that you didn't eat enough proteins and vegetables for dinner. If you feel hungrier at four p.m., before dinner, then you probably didn't eat enough proteins and vegetables for lunch. Pay close attention to what you ate earlier. You notice that you might need to double your portion size if you're eating fish or chicken. Make a mental note or write it down so that you remember to eat more of that dish the next time in order to avoid feeling hungry or to develop cravings.

Rather than tracking your emotions, track your hunger and cravings. For example, it's common to resort to "comfort" foods to soothe your anxiety when you're feeling stressed out. Instead of eating cookies or pasta, pick foods that won't spike your insulin level such as pickles, flame-broiled chicken, or steak. These are only examples. The idea is to eat foods that won't spike your insulin level to make you feel full and happy. If you're full after eating a juicy steak, you're less likely to want pasta or sweets.

Another self-monitoring technique is regular weighing. It's best to weigh yourself once a week rather than daily, as day-to-day fluctuations aren't good indicators of your actual weight. Throughout Thinsulin, keeping track of your weight is important. During the Active Phase, if you notice that you're stuck on the same weight for two weeks, examine what you ate so that you can identify the foods that might be raising your insulin level. It's also very important to weigh yourself during the Passive Phase. If you maintain your weight, you're doing great. If you notice that you've gained more than five pounds, you'll need to go back to the Active Phase.

At 5′ and 210.4 pounds (BMI of 41), Norma, thirty-four, came to Lorphen Medical to lose weight because she wasn't able to keep up with her three children ranging from six to eighteen years old. She tried to eat healthier on her own but she wasn't able to lose weight.

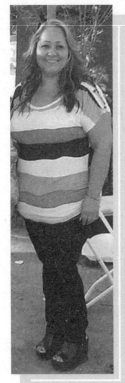

Norma Before:
March 2015,
210.4 pounds

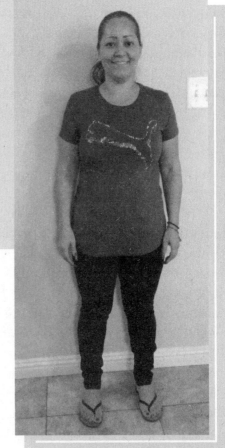

Norma After: October 2015,
146.4 pounds

After seven months on the Thinsulin Program, she lost 64 pounds, or 30.4 percent of her initial weight.

Norma shared that coming to Lorphen Medical weekly to weigh in helps her stay on track. If her weight remains unchanged for a few weeks, she reviews what she ate and tries to understand what foods might have spike her insulin level. With the help of Dr. Charles T. Nguyen, she's able to make necessary adjustments to her food choices, allowing her body to lose weight again.

In short, self-monitoring is an important aspect of behavioral modification. There are many ways of doing it. It's up to you whether or not you want to keep a food log or journal or whether you want to write it down in a notebook or use online programs. You need to monitor your hunger and cravings daily, and your weight weekly. While self-monitoring provides you with the awareness, you need to translate this knowledge into actions that will change your behavior.

FEEDBACK AND REINFORCEMENT

As we go back to how habits are changed, we see the importance of feedback as a positive or negative reinforcement. As you plug away through your weight-loss journey, you'll receive plenty of feedback (whether you want it or not!). Your friends, neighbors, coworkers, or physician will notice your weight loss. They often will compliment you and then offer you their own piece of advice. However, a lot of times, their well-intentioned guidance might contradict what you've learned. They might encourage you to cheat during the weekends or tell you that it's OK to just have the smallest bite of a cookie. They might tell you tales of how they were able to lose weight in the past. As you know, it's very difficult to give up bad habits. It doesn't get any easier to break bad habits if you cheat.

In your journey, accept the compliments that can serve as powerful reinforcement to motivate you to continue. However, process the suggestions offered to make sure it doesn't conflict with what you've learned. If you're unable to lose weight, don't beat yourself up. You'll have to put weight loss in perspective. While weight loss will make you healthier, it doesn't guarantee you a happier marriage, a better job, or higher grades. Don't fall into the magical thinking that weight loss will solve all your problems. That's the unrealistic expectation that will only set you up for disappointment.

Instead, focus on whether or not you're spiking your insulin with every meal. Visualize in your mind how insulin would spike if you eat that cake. As you see your insulin rising, you understand that your body will reverse course and now store rather than burn fat. Knowing that it takes three weeks to bring down insulin again, ask yourself, "Is it really worth it to cheat with that cookie?" If you choose to walk away, this will serve as positive reinforcement because you're able to overcome your weakness. On the other hand, if you end up eating the cookie, the mere fact that you've wasted all your effort may serve as negative reinforcement to help you change as well.

It's similar to wearing braces to straighten your teeth. The initial process can be painful as the dentist might have to extract several teeth before the orthodontist can put on braces. Month after month, you would return to the office to have your wires readjusted. Throughout this time, you would endure the pain, the inconvenience of being unable to eat solid foods, and the annoyance of having food stuck in your braces. But after several years, you finally achieve your goal of having a beautiful smile when your braces are removed. As you know very well, this is not the end. You still have to wear a retainer every night if you want to keep your teeth straight. If you don't, your teeth will slowly migrate back to their crooked position.

In summary, you can break bad habits and form healthier ones by using these techniques. You must always be on the lookout and practice what you've learned. Bad habits often return if you don't pay attention, and if you deviate from the program. We're confident that you'll be able to break your bad habits. We know that you can give up eating before you go to bed or opting to eat candy after a stressful day. The Thinsulin Program gives you the power to exert control over your life. You'll learn how to control your cravings in the next chapter.

Chapter 15

CONTROLLING FOOD CRAVINGS

We all have food cravings. One study showed that an astonishing 97 percent of women and 68 percent of men reported episodes of food cravings. To add another rung to the ladder, there's temptation *everywhere*. You've got cookies in your pantry, chips at a friend's house, and chocolate treats at work. Some, if not all, of these foods are screaming for you to eat them. They even seem to know your name. Realistically, how can you walk away?

The traditional approach tells you to ignore your food cravings. This simply doesn't work! You struggle to stay away from junk food for a few days, only to relent after a stressful day at work by downing the chocolate cake. If you're unable to walk away from your cravings, you berate yourself for lacking self-control and willpower.

Rule number one: Don't feel bad if you succumb to your cravings. It happens even when you're not aware of it. A study published in the *Journal of the American Dietetic Association* showed that *unconscious* neurobehavioral processes in the brain drive people to crave and overeat, rather than a lack of willpower or self-control. What can you do to fight the cravings?

By understanding the "why" rather than just the "how," you'll gain new insight to help you beat your cravings. We'll first discuss the processes of food reward, inhibitory control, and time discounting to help you understand that cravings are actually "hard-wired" in your brain. Then, we'll teach you how to overcome these hard-wired brain processes in order to control your food cravings.

FOOD REWARD

The Science: The brain harbors a reward system. When we pursue pleasurable foods, the brain rewards us by making us feel good. People can fall prey to overeating and other addictions if our reward circuit is oversensitive. Sugar has a profound effect on the brain reward system.

Princeton University's Dr. Bart Hoebel showed that rats that were denied and then reintroduced to sugar developed craving and relapse behaviors as they consumed more sugar. The researchers restricted the rats' food while they slept and for four hours after waking, so that the rats were hungry. This echoes people skipping breakfast. The rats were then allowed to eat and drink sugar water, a phenomenon known as sugar-bingeing. After a month, the researchers found that the rats' brain structures adapted to the increased dopamine levels, leading to fewer dopamine receptors, while showing more opioid receptors. In other words, sugar was shown to provoke surges in dopamine and opioid levels under certain circumstances, which can be a sign of addiction. The changes seen in these rat studies are also seen in the brains of rats on cocaine and heroin. Furthermore, when the rats' sugar supply was removed, their brain levels of dopamine dropped, leading to worsening anxiety, teeth chattering, and an unwillingness to venture forth into the open arm of the maze. Normally, rats like to explore their environment, but rats in sugar withdrawal were too anxious to explore, preferring instead to stay in a tunnel area.

The Solution: No cheating on sweets such as desserts, snacks, or drinks. As long as you continue to feed your brain's reward system with sugar, you'll have a heck of a tough time getting rid of your cravings. The true solution is to cleanse your system of sugar and sugar substitutes in order to extinguish your sugar cravings. Any weight-loss programs that allow "cheating" with sweets don't take into account these powerful neurobehavioral processes. This explains why the failure rates of many diets are so high. How can you control your sugar cravings if you continue to feed them? Cheating with sweets only reinforces your brain circuitry to want more sugar. Don't sabotage yourself right out of the gate.

INHIBITORY CONTROL

The Science: It's widely believed that the prefrontal cortex part of the brain is the source of the inhibitory control process, which in turn helps control eating impulses. Research has shown that people with weaker inhibitory control are often obese, eat more high-calorie food, and are unsuccessful in trying to lose weight than those with more effective inhibitory control. In other words, people with poor inhibitory control are more likely to succumb to temptations and indulge in foods rich in calories. Unfortunately, we all have poor inhibitory control because of normal stressors in life. When we all feel bummed out, we tend to resort to food that comforts us. When we feel stressed out, we might turn to food to relieve our distress. Therefore, it's important to manage stress in order to overcome the poor inhibitory control.

The Solution: No starving. While you can't control normal life stressors, you certainly can learn to control your eating habits. By skipping meals or starving yourself, you'll only add more unnecessary stress to your body. So it's important to eat five times a day. Eat more often—not less! Eating breakfast will help you prepare for the day. The morning snack with a low-GI fruit will help you satisfy the sugar craving while providing enough energy to last until lunch. Eating enough green, leafy vegetables and at least one portion or more of protein for lunch will power you through the afternoon. The afternoon snack of a portion of nuts will bridge the time between lunch and dinner. Of course, a dinner consisting of green, leafy vegetables and at least one portion or more of protein will ensure that you have enough nutrients and energy to last throughout the night. Any time that you feel hungry or you crave carbs or sweets is a sign that you didn't eat enough protein for lunch or dinner. Try your best to eat five times a day in order to minimize the amount of stress on your body.

It's Murphy's Law that there'll be times you'll be bummed out by some terrible news or things won't go your way. It's easy to resort to pleasurable foods to perk you up. When this happens, we want you to stop for a minute and identify your emotions. If you recognize your feelings and acknowledge the emotion, you can address the real issue instead of turning to your comfort food. A study in the *Journal of Marketing Research* found that people who have a better understanding of their feelings were more likely to pick healthier options and lose more weight than those who aren't in touch with their feelings, regardless of how much they previously knew about nutrition. So, the next time you have a bad day, don't just blow it off. Confide in someone about how you feel. This may prevent you from cheating on some chips or sweets. Of course, if you eat enough to feel full, this will also minimize the risk of succumbing to your cravings.

TIME DISCOUNTING

The Science: The third neurobehavioral process that contributes to craving is time discounting. This involves the mesolimbic system and prefrontal cortex. Your brain wants something now rather than later, especially when it comes to food. If someone offers you a piece of pie, it's hard to say no and take it home to eat later. Your brain creates an intense desire for you to eat the pie immediately. If you pass on it, you may develop intense cravings for it, think about it all day, and stop by a grocery or corner bakery to satisfy your craving. We realize we're describing this with drug or alcohol overtones, but according to the study we mentioned above, there are direct similarities.

The solution: Change your thinking. It's easy to fall prey to thinking that nursing a craving means you're doomed to relapse or that you're unmotivated. Understand that it's not your fault. Again, it's common to have cravings, especially because now you understand the neurobehavioral processes. When your brain tells you to want something N-O-W, it's difficult to resist by simply walking away.

Again, that's why it's so important to always pause and think in terms of insulin. If you're tempted to eat what's in front of you, ask yourself if it will spike your insulin level. If it does, what will happen? Your body will store fat without burning fat. How long does it take to lower your insulin level again? Three weeks. Not one. Not two. Three. So, is it worth it to eat it? If you think it's worth it, do it. If you don't lose weight, you'll understand exactly why. And that's OK. If you did succumb to your cravings, you didn't do anything wrong! The food can really hit the spot. You see, what we're trying to do here is to remove the good-versus-bad, right-versus-wrong, punishment-versus-reward thinking often associated with dieting. By learning to assess these situations neutrally instead, you gain control over your cravings. The question simply becomes, will the food increase your insulin level or not? And you already know the answer.

While it's helpful to challenge your cravings by thinking in terms of insulin, the best way to fight your cravings is to play defense. Don't put yourself in a situation where you'll fall prey to the cravings. Think ahead and prepare your meals for the next day. It doesn't mean that you must pack your food for lunch or cook your dinners, although this can be helpful. It means that you need to anticipate where you're going and plan what you're going to have. If it's a new restaurant, check the online menu beforehand for favorite foods that won't spike your insulin level.

We get how tough it is to fight food cravings. That's why we want you to take it one day at a time. Slowly, over time, you'll find it easier and easier to shrug off certain foods. A study involving two hundred seventy men and women found that, over time, restricting specific types of food might decrease food cravings. So, it'll get easier.

If you still find it difficult to fight cravings, you may want to talk to your physician to see if a prescription-weight loss medication—along with diet and exercise—is right for you. You'll find detailed information on medications in Appendix A.

Chapter 16

A NEW BEGINNING

By now, you undoubtedly see the connection between insulin and weight loss. We've shared with you a novel approach of merging medicine with psychiatry to create a powerfully simple and effective weight management program. You've read many research studies and gained more insight into the biopsychosocial concept to help you lose weight and keep it off.

Sugar as it relates to weight gain is not a new concept, with the focus placed squarely on calories associated with sweets. But Thinsulin shifts the focus away from calories toward insulin. By teaching you to think in terms of insulin, you free your mind from the constraints of dieting and allow yourself the opportunity for meaningful, lifelong changes.

Thousands and growing numbers of people have had success with the Thinsulin Program. Here's one more story of one patient's dramatic weight-loss success on the program:

Joanne, a sixty-year-old housewife from Southern California, had undergone many diet programs in her life. During life's worst stressors, she often packed on pounds. In the past, she would turn to obsessive exercise to burn off the calories when she gained a lot of weight. She would spend three to four hours a day (!) doing hardcore aerobics, jumping from one class to another in order to lose weight. The more she worked out, the more stress she put on her arthritic knees. She was obsessed with burning calories. At her addiction's worst, she would augment these classes with up to eleven cycle classes weekly and three to four hours of weightlifting a day. She paid a huge price to get her weight down: the osteoarthritis in her knees was so bad it was too painful to walk. She was also plagued with daily migraines.

When Joanne was physically unable to exercise, she gained back her weight because she wasn't able to burn off all the calories she ate. Like many dieters, her weight fluctuated with operatic drama. As soon as her pain improved, she was back at the gym, only to be shut down again due to her knees.

She knew she couldn't keep this up. Her weight peaked at 189 pounds in the fall of 2011. At Joanne's height of 5′2″, her BMI was 34.6. But her weight really hit home when she saw her photo from her daughter's graduation. Wearing a pumpkin-colored dress to the celebration party that evening, she remembered vividly what her daughter said to her: "Mom, you look like an orange tent." Those seven jaw-dropping, life-changing words led her to seek out a weight-loss program.

Joanne thought Weight Watchers® would be a good fit because it primarily focuses on calories rather than on exercise. However, after a few weekly sessions, she became obsessed with their point system, often starving or bingeing as a result. To avoid embarrassment at the weekly weigh-in, she'd push herself with increasing intensity.

At the weigh-ins, people line up behind a screen to get on the scale. Joanne would get stressed out because she didn't want people to know that she hadn't lost weight. She didn't want to share with the group afterward what went wrong, or if she had been weak and unmotivated. "I so feared public shame that beforehand I would take off my bra and glasses, empty my bladder, and make sure I'd starved myself plenty," she says.

Even though Weight Watchers® can be a supportive environment, Joanne couldn't help but feel humiliation. "I think avoiding public embarrassment in front of my peers at the weigh-ins added to my obsessive behavior," she explains. She would diligently count her points and watch her portions. She received so much adoration and support for her weight loss, fueling her quest to eat even less so that she would continue to do what she had to do—however unhealthy she knew it to be—to continue to lose pounds. And lose weight she did—too much weight. Her weight careened so low—to 121 pounds—that her doctor warned her she would have a heart attack if she didn't stop starving herself. "He told me I was killing myself," says Joanne. "I had to listen."

Joanne stopped keeping track of the points and watching her portion size. As a result, she slowly gained weight over time. She also dropped the weekly Weight Watchers® meeting because she didn't want to explain to her peers why she was gaining weight. She didn't want to feel that same pressure again. But eventually, she had to do something about her weight once more as it crept up to 171 pounds in April 2014. Her daily migraines had returned as well. She didn't want to return to her all-time high of 189 pounds.

When Joanne learned about the Thinsulin Program offered at Lorphen Medical, she knew this was different. Counter to the conventional wisdom regarding weight loss, she was surprised to learn about the primary role insulin plays. All her life, she was told that she needed to eat less and exercise more. Yet she hadn't been able to conquer the endless loop of dieting and the dreaded yo-yo effect. She put her soul into this very different weight-loss program. "I'm a twenty-year cancer survivor," she says today. "I'm a fighter!"

Joanne lamented on what she'd learned about nutrition in the past. "We aren't taught that lowering insulin is why we lose weight," she says incredulously. "Or about the relationship between sugar, calories, and insulin. Even when I had cancer, no one—doctors or nurses—told me that cancer feeds on sugar."

Thinsulin goes far beyond sugar. Even if sugar-free or artificial sweeteners don't affect your insulin level, they'll cause you to crave sweets later on, making you more prone to cheating.

Like many, Joanne was surprised to learn this. To start, she had to undo the false belief that she was out of harm's way in drinking *sugar-free* creamer. In fact, she drank 64 ounces of coffee with sugar-free

French Vanilla creamer a day. To kill her sugar cravings, she had to get rid of all sweets, especially the artificial sweeteners. Joanne was asked to drink water, unsweetened iced tea, or black coffee. "At first, I thought, there's no way I can do this," Joanne remembered. But, she said, "Within 24 hours, I didn't have any more migraines!" While there isn't a documented correlation between drinking black coffee and being headache-free, Joanne's experience enabled her to give up creamer, knowing that she would no longer suffer from the horrific, daily migraines that had plagued her previously.

Until Thinsulin, she hadn't realized how many carbs and sweets she had been eating regularly. After one week on Thinsulin, Joanne dropped 7 pounds. After one month, she lost 16.2 pounds or 9.5 percent of her weight. Suddenly she found that she no longer craved sweets. "My morning fruit satisfies me," she said. The afternoon snack of raw nuts consistently helped to keep her full until dinner. Joanne was able to go out with her friends and family to different restaurants and try new dishes. "I just think in terms of insulin," she said simply. "I feel like I'm in control again. Food doesn't control me!"

For too long, Joanne felt helpless when it came to her weight. She didn't like feeling out of control by seeing her weight drop, only to see it rebound again. She thought she either had to starve or exert herself to lose weight. None of what she did taught her how to keep the weight off long term.

Thinsulin offered an alternative solution. Its low-pressure, no-calorie-counting, flexible system helped her learn "how to fish" in her weight-loss journey. "In Weight Watchers®, if you use your points and you're starving, then you don't eat, or else you cheat," says Joanne. "With Thinsulin, you eat five times a day. You don't starve yourself. It's not stressful. There's no pressure."

Not only was she able to lose weight, but as of June 2015, she's maintaining her weight at 132.6 pounds, which is a normal BMI of 24.3. "In the Passive Phase, I can have my enjoyment foods in the morning and work them off during the day," she says with enthusiasm.

Thinsulin works well for Joanne, and it can work well for you. In the end, Thinsulin transformed Joanne into a more confident person who's able to regain control of her weight, and most important, her entire life.

And that orange dress? Gone. "To remind myself how far I've come, I reward myself by buying a new dress every Tuesday," she says with a laugh.

———————

One reason we created the Thinsulin Program is because we're facing a growing worldwide obesity epidemic that threatens the health of our current and future generations. We need novel approaches and a paradigm shift from what we're currently offering if we want to win this battle against obesity. We can't simply resort to quick fixes alone, or expect lifestyle changes without offering a program that addresses the biology of insulin to burn fat, psychology of CBT to change your thinking, and behavioral modifications to break habits.

My brother and I both have the same mission of fighting the obesity epidemic, but our different medical training and expertise set the stage for us to create this breakthrough weight-loss program. The synergy between the working of the body and the power of the mind will transform your life. By tapping into the depths of your complex weight issues, the Thinsulin Program challenges your current thought process, and ultimately, changes your behavior and eating habits. We've seen thousands of people succeed with the Thinsulin Program. Like Joanne and the others you've met in this book, you will, too.

It's been over thirty-six years since our parents embarked on an amazing journey to give my brother, two other siblings, and me an opportunity to pursue the American Dream by leaving our ancestral homeland on a small fishing boat. We're humbled by this experience and so grateful for a new beginning. We wish to give back so that others may enjoy the opportunities we're so blessed to have.

We truly believe the Thinsulin Program will revolutionize the way you think about obesity, in terms of insulin rather than calories. We dream of one day where you can go to restaurants that offer a Thinsulin menu, knowing that the foods you eat won't spike your insulin level during the Active Phase, and minimize your insulin spike during the Passive Phase. By sharing the concepts of Thinsulin, we believe this is the paradigm shift that will win and reverse the obesity epidemic.

So put your past away, and set sail for a new beginning. Instead of a small fishing boat, you'll be traveling in a large yacht filled with immeasurable knowledge and renewed motivation. We wish you the best of luck on your journey.

FREQUENTLY ASKED QUESTIONS

We want to take the opportunity to answer the most popular questions we're asked regarding Thinsulin, weight loss, and staying healthy. Here's to knowing better and doing better!

MAY I DRINK ALCOHOL?

For those who drink socially, one of the difficulties of going on a diet is to give up alcohol altogether. Although ideal, it's not always realistic. The good news is, it's possible to still drink alcohol and not increase your insulin significantly. Just keep it to one drink.

Some people blame the calories for the "beer belly," but it's really about the insulin. They may cite the fact that a light beer contains only 96 calories and 3.2 grams of carbohydrates while a regular beer contains 150 calories and 13 grams of carbohydrates. Your caloric intake is less with light beers, but the potential for insulin spike is still there. You see, beers are made from grains such as wheat or barley. These grains still spike insulin level, causing the body to store fat. Where else? You guessed it. Right in your gut. That's why you'll see a "beer belly" on someone who likes to indulge regularly in a cold one.

Have you ever seen a "wine belly"? Not really, right? That's because wine is made from fermented grapes, a low-GI fruit. As long as you drink one glass of wine, it won't necessarily spike your insulin level. That's why you don't see a "wine belly."

White wine has fewer calories than red wine. A 5-ounce glass of red wine typically contains 150 calories and 5 grams of carbohydrates, while a 5-ounce glass of white wine contains about 84 calories and 3 grams of carbohydrates. Avoid drinking dessert wine such as ice wine as it may spike your insulin level. Each drop of ice wine is squeezed from one grape. You can imagine how many grapes go into a 5-ounce glass and its resulting effect on insulin.

You can drink hard liquor such as vodka, rum, whiskey, gin, and tequila, even though they are *distilled* from the fermentation of potatoes, sugarcane, grained mashes (barley, rye, wheat, and corn), juniper berries, and agave plants, respectively. Wait a minute! You may ponder why it's OK to drink these hard liquors made from grains, potatoes, and sugarcanes. The distillation process results in ethyl alcohol, which is eventually broken down by the liver into acetate, and finally into carbon dioxide and water. It doesn't result in sugar, so the GI for hard liquor is zero. It simply won't spike your insulin level if you drink it on the rocks or by itself. Don't do mixed drinks with other sugary drinks such as cranberries or orange juice. Cocktails with vodka as the main ingredient, such as a Bloody Mary, Screwdriver, Sex on the Beach, and Black or White Russian, will definitely spike your insulin level. The same can be said for the rum found in mojitos, piña coladas, and mai tais.

IS THINSULIN SIMILAR TO A LOW-CARB DIET LIKE ATKINS OR PALEO?

What do low-carb diets such as Paleo and Atkins mean to you? From the name, it must mean the foods are low in carbohydrates. That's not completely accurate. While low-carb diets encourage high-protein intake, they also contain foods that are actually high in carbohydrates. This may be contrary to your understanding. We'll explain more by examining the Paleo and Atkins diets in detail.

The Paleolithic diet, more commonly known as the Paleo diet, mimics the diet of our ancient hunter and gatherer ancestors. The idea is to eat a large proportion of meat, raw fruits, and vegetables. On the Paleo diet, you can have leafy greens such as spinach, arugula, kale, and mixed baby greens. You may also have monosaturated fats and oils such as nuts, seeds, and avocados. You can have berries and beets. Of course, you can have plenty of lean meat, seafood, and eggs.

The Atkins diet became popular worldwide after Dr. Robert C. Atkins wrote the best-selling book in 1972. The Atkins diet consists of four different phases. The initial induction phase of Atkins is the strictest phase. It permits 20 grams of carbohydrates in the form of green, leafy vegetables such as spinach, broccoli, and asparagus. The next phase is the balancing phase. This is when you slowly add more nuts and a small amount of fruits back into your diet. The third phase, called the fine-tuning phase, is characterized by adding even more carbohydrates to your diet. The last phase is the maintenance phase, where you can eat healthy carbohydrates while trying to maintain your weight. It's similar to the Passive Phase of Thinsulin.

Some people choose to skip the induction phase by adding fruits to the diet early on, while others choose to stay in the induction phase for a long period of time. This is sometimes called the ketogenic diet because it restricts carbohydrate intake.

In both diets, you're still allowed to eat green, leafy vegetables. As you recall from reading about carbohydrates in Chapter 5, these vegetables are actually cellulose or polysaccharides. Polysaccharides are made of thousands of glucose linked together by beta bonds, which can't be broken down by humans. Therefore, the green, leafy vegetables stay largely intact during digestion, without releasing any glucose. They are considered fiber or cellulose. More important, they don't spike the insulin level.

As you can see, it's not accurate to say that the Atkins and Paleo diet are low-carb diets when, in fact, they allow eating a lot of carbohydrates such as green, leafy vegetables. It's more accurate to say that these diets minimize the spike in insulin level.

ARE ALL SPARKLING WATERS THE SAME?

A good alternative to drinking soda is switching to sparkling water. Sparkling water is produced through a carbonation process where carbon dioxide gas is dissolved in water to create tiny bubbles or gas. All sparkling water is calorie free. Yet just because it has the word "water," doesn't mean all sparkling waters are the same.

Mineral Water

Sparkling mineral water comes from a natural spring or well. No minerals or carbonation are added to the water. The bubbles and minerals such as salt and sulfur compounds arise organically from a natural spring, so there are no added chemicals.

Club Soda and Seltzer Water

These are both very similar as they are made with plain water artificially carbonated. Club soda is different from Seltzer water because minerals such as potassium bicarbonate are added to the club soda to enhance the flavor. Seltzer water gets its name from the German town of Selters, which is known for its natural springs.

Tonic Water

Tonic water is carbonated and contains a little quinine to give it a bitter taste. Sugar, typically HFCS, is added to minimize the bitter taste, along with other spices. Therefore, tonic water will spike your insulin level and should be avoided. Unlike all carbonated water, it contains about 130 calories for 12 fluid ounces.

The bottom line is that carbonated water is a good alternative to water. Except for tonic water, it contains no calories or sugar. It hydrates like plain water. If you miss the caffeine or bubbly taste of a soda, you can put a bag of brewed tea into your carbonated water along with a slice of lemon to give it a great taste. You get the caffeine from the tea and bubbles from the carbonated water, but no calories that you would typically get with sodas.

MAY I ADD SPICES AND HERBS TO FOODS?

Remember, the Thinsulin Program isn't a diet. You don't ever have to eat bland foods—you get to enjoy your foods. It's OK for it to taste good! Feel free to add any herbs and spices to your dish. You don't need to worry so much about the effects on insulin unless you're drowning your dish with them. Spices such as cayenne pepper, cinnamon, garlic, turmeric, ginger, ginseng, and mustard seed can add flavor to your meat dish without causing your insulin to spike. You can use all types of herbs as well to marinade your meat dish or add to your spaghetti sauce.

Just be careful when you're cooking. Some recipes specify using brown or white sugar. Don't add them as these may spike your insulin level. Other spices will make up for the flavor.

Likewise, be very careful when you're marinating your fish or meat. If possible, use fresh spices and herbs to marinate it simply because you know exactly what you're using. Be careful about using a pre-marinated sauce that you buy at the store or buying marinated meat ready for cooking. Oftentimes, it contains a lot of brown sugar. That explains the brown residue stuck on the grill.

HOW DO I PREPARE MY VEGETABLES?

When it comes to eating vegetables, you have many ways to prepare them. You don't always have to eat your vegetables raw or as salads. Leafy vegetables such as arugula, lettuce, and spinach can be eaten raw, with Italian or balsamic and vinaigrette dressing on the side (if using bottled dressing, be sure it doesn't contain added sugar), along with other vegetables that won't spike the insulin level. Just make sure you don't add potatoes, corn, carrots, or beets to your salad. Kale can be a bit more difficult to make. By itself, kale is rather bitter, but if you add lemon juice along with garlic as a dressing, the acid from the lemon "cooks" the kale, making it rather tasty. Try to add vegetables with high fiber (kale, spinach, or celery) to your salad. Lettuce is low in fiber, so you may still have constipation despite eating a ton of lettuce.

You can boil or steam your vegetables. Sure, you're not adding oil but don't worry so much that your food becomes bland. Make sure you add garlic or other spices to make your vegetables delicious. Consider steaming the celery roots and make mashed celery as a replacement for mashed potatoes; mashed cauliflower also makes a nice alternative. You can always blend celery or asparagus into a hearty soup. Yes, it won't taste exactly the same as mashed potatoes but if you spice it correctly, it can come pretty close.

You can also roast your vegetables. Chop up your favorite vegetables, add a little olive oil and spices. Use the juice from the roasted chicken to flavor your roasted broccoli or asparagus. You can even bake the kale into chips. Just wash the kale, sprinkle some salt, and bake it to perfection. Imagine how that would taste with some fresh salsa?

If you're craving Chinese food, you can sauté or stir-fry your vegetables. Add some soy sauce, garlic, onions, and other spices to add flavor. Make sure you use olive or vegetable oil, not corn oil, to stir-fry your vegetables. Some recipes call for adding cornstarch to thicken the sauce. Stop and think before you proceed. Adding cornstarch (corn is a vegetable and starch already gives it away) will definitely spike your insulin level. Use oyster sauce in moderation as it contains sugar as well.

If you're in the mood for grilling, you can brush the vegetables with olive oil, add your favorite seasoning, and grill them along with your chicken, fish, or beef. Be creative and grill different vegetables. Just make sure you're not picking any vegetables that would spike your insulin level.

Similar to your vegetables, you have many options to prepare your chicken, beef, fish, or other seafood. It all depends on your taste. Whether you choose to steam your fish, grill your chicken, stir-fry your beef, or roast your turkey, make sure you add spices and herbs to make it taste good. Remember, you're not on a diet, so make sure you enjoy what you eat!

ARE VEGETARIANS ABLE TO DO THINSULIN?

Absolutely. Vegetarians can be completely successful on the Thinsulin Program. You just have to be creative to stay within the concepts of insulin. Instead of getting protein from meat, vegetarians will get protein from plants, including soy products, nuts, beans, and dairy products. Ovo-vegetarians may consume eggs, but not dairy products, while lacto-vegetarians avoid eggs while consuming dairy products. Vegans abstain from any animal products, including eggs and dairy products. A study published in the *British Journal of Medicine* showed a low-carbohydrate, plant-based diet called the "Eco-Atkins" diet to result in weight loss and improvement in cholesterol.

It may not seem like you have that many choices for your protein. That's not exactly true. You have to look around and find recipes that fit your taste. Don't eat the same thing every day. Make sure you eat enough protein to keep you full. Whatever you do, don't make your food bland.

Meat substitutes such as Quorn™ products are high in protein. They are made from Mycoprotein, through a fermentation process from a fungus called *Fusarium venenatum*. It's a healthy protein source that is high in fiber but low in saturated fat. You can add Quorn™ mince, Quorn™ meat-free chicken pieces, and Quorn™ standard sausages as meat substitutes to your breakfast, lunch, or dinner.

Many vegetarian dishes use seitan, a meat substitute derived from wheat gluten. Be careful of eating seitan if you're allergic to gluten. Consider soy products instead because soy is less likely to spike insulin.

Soy products are a great source of your protein. You can buy the Wildwood products such as the meatless crumbles to make tacos (without the shells) or meatballs to add to your squash spaghetti. Soy burgers are less likely to spike insulin compared with other veggie burgers that are made from grains. Don't just depend on soy products as your only source of protein.

Beans would also make good protein alternatives, but try to minimize their intake as they do contain carbohydrates. Some are more likely to spike insulin than others. Beans that have fewer carbohydrates include lima, fava, great Northern, mung, lentils, black-eyed peas, and green peas.

Depending on your preferences, you can also add egg whites or dairy products to provide enough protein to keep you full. Of course, make sure you eat more green, leafy vegetables. The high fiber will help keep you full as well.

Are Vegetarians Able to Do Thinsulin?

Sephira, a patient at Lorphen Medical Clinic in Riverside, California, lost a total of 60 pounds on Thinsulin. Here's her story in her own words:

I took a 40-year journey to lose 60 pounds. I weighed an unhealthy 189 when I began seeing Dr. Charles T. Nguyen on May 22, 2013. At a mere 5'3", this put my BMI at 33.5, considered expressly obese.

I was overweight throughout my childhood. As a kid, my parents fed me unhealthy breakfasts that included sugary cereal, donuts, ice cream or cookies; sandwiches, chips, cookies, and soda for lunch and fast food meals that usually consisted of hamburgers, French fries, soda, and ice cream for dinner. Having junk food-addicted parents and a father who controlled all of the finances, we ate what he told us to buy. I was called names as most overweight children are, and was even teased by my own father, who was obese himself. My parents never sought help for me. I was determined to have a healthier lifestyle when I moved out of my parents' house. I soon found that I was addicted to all of the unhealthy foods my parents were. By the age of twenty, I weighed 160 pounds.

Then the popular combination of diet pills, fen-phen, was launched—and I had to try it. Finally, success! I lost 35 pounds in three months. I went back to my high school weight of 125 pounds! I kept the weight off for three and a half years, but then I began working a desk job for a major corporation. Between working and commuting I was sitting for thirteen hours a day, and the weight began to creep up over the next fourteen years. My weight went up and down—mostly up.

My weight increased to 195 pounds. When dieting didn't work, I fasted. I drank water only and ate once every three days. I was so desperate that I got down to 167 in one month. I began dating the man who is now my husband and started eating again. I became pregnant, was very sick, lost weight, and then packed on 55 pounds.

After getting married and moving to a different job in 2006, the weight began to creep up again. I decided to become a vegetarian. I thought that was going to help my weight, too. Wrong! My weight had shot up again by May of 2013. I felt like the odds were against me.

Soon before my thirty-eighth birthday, I decided enough was enough. My health issues were worse than ever. I was out on FMLA (the Family and Medical Leave Act, which allowed me to take time off for medical reasons) for chronic migraines, and I started to believe that my issues could be due to the abuse I endured growing up. Perhaps my weight was my protection, and I subconsciously kept it on. After all, there was just no reason for my obesity. All of my blood tests came back normal. Now what?

I began researching weight-loss doctors and programs. I was limited because I'm allergic to prepackaged foods, nor did I want injections or surgery, and I'd already failed at counting points and eating a low-carb, high-fat diet. A new weight-loss clinic had opened up near my house so I decided to look at their website. I was immediately intrigued, but disliked doctors because of unpleasant experiences, so I was hesitant. I decided to send Dr. Charles T. Nguyen an email to see what he had to say about my lack of weight-loss success. The response I received was immediate and unexpected. He nicely offered very useful information that I had never heard before. It was time to schedule an appointment.

I was greeted with kindness, professionalism and encouragement—and have been ever since. I have never been rushed or talked down to. Everything he has taught me has always made sense and has been easy to understand. I learned to think differently about food—just as he said!

By the ninth week on Thinsulin, I had lost 19 pounds, and it showed! I had dropped four sizes! I couldn't believe it! The puffiness in my body had started to go away, my skin looked clearer, and people noticed! I was hooked! Dr. Nguyen had the key to my weight loss and I was happy to unlock the benefits.

After losing more weight, I experienced my first "Big Moment." I went to my favorite department store to try on the designer jeans that I had wanted so desperately to fit into. I had no idea what size I wore. For fun, I grabbed a pair of size 30 jeans. I thought maybe I would get them over my thighs, but I was not counting on it because they make these jeans for skinny girls, not for chunky girls like me. I tried on other sizes first and to my amazement, they were all too big! Jeans are never too big, always too small when I try them on. I slowly put on the size 30s—over my calves, over my thighs, and I kept trying them on in total disbelief that they were fitting. Next, I pulled them over my buttocks and buttoned them easily. I was in shock, so I checked the tags because this could not be right. Nope, these are a size 30, a size I never wore before and I am wearing them! *Me!* After all the "oh my Gods," I cried in that dressing room. Full-blown crying, tears ruining my makeup. I had to take a picture and send it to my husband. It wasn't real unless someone else was seeing this, too! I continued to lose weight on the Thinsulin Program. In August 2014, nearly fifteen months after I saw Dr. Nguyen, I had lost 60 pounds, dropping 32 percent of my weight. I went from being obese (BMI of 33.5) to having a normal weight (BMI of 22.9).

I was a real person with a success story!

Aside from being able to wear clothes I never thought I would fit into, I felt better! I had more energy, felt happier, was excited to get

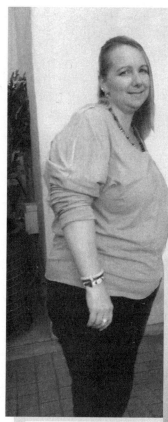

Sephira Before:
May 2013, 189 pounds

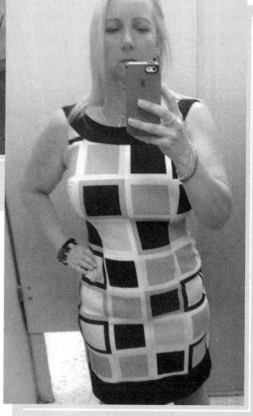

Sephira After:
August 2014, 129 pounds

dressed in the morning. Fashion excited me once again. I was comfortable in my own skin for the first time in my entire life. I felt confidence that I had never felt before. Instead of worrying that people would be judging me on my size, I was worried they were judging me on my fashion sense! Which, by the way, I am not gifted with. I had been taking cues from my coworkers, who were quick to tell me that my pants were too baggy and that I was clueless to what my actual size was! Even now, I have to be reminded sometimes that I'm not "fat" anymore and to stop dressing like I am. That was a serious reality check!

DOES EATING LATE LEAD TO WEIGHT GAIN?

Sometimes, you don't have control over your work schedule. An emergency can spring up out of nowhere, causing you to stay at work longer than you anticipated. When you get home, it might be so late that you're afraid to eat dinner because of the potential weight gain. You heard that you burn more calories during the day, so it's not good to eat late at night because the late-night calories sit in your body and turn into fat.

Let's dispel this myth.

The reality is, calories can't tell time. Your body will use the calories the same way whether it's early in the morning or late at night. It really depends on what you're eating. Just make sure that what you're eating won't spike insulin. Everything goes back to this simple rule. It's better to have your dinner late than to skip it altogether. If you skip, you'll find that you're going to feel very hungry the next day, and you'll end up overeating.

If you already had dinner and still feel hungry, then eating a late-night snack will definitely lead to weight gain. Oftentimes, night eaters eat not because they're hungry, but because they want to satisfy their cravings to cope with stress or boredom. Research shows that many women take in nearly half of their daily calories at or after dinner. That's a lot of calories! That's why it's important to eat enough protein at dinner so that you feel full. You're less likely to snack if you're full.

HOW WOULD I DO THINSULIN
IF I WORK THE NIGHT SHIFT?

We have numerous shift workers in our program. Many of them work night shifts as dispatchers, police officers, or nurses. They often work for three to four nights in a row, and then they have to get back to their normal schedule. The adjustments can be difficult. Not getting enough sleep affects their appetite. Sometimes, they don't feel hungry at all. When they skip meals, they find themselves so hungry later on that they would have to eat a huge meal to satisfy their hunger. The difficulty is in trying to fit in five meals when their sleep changes once or twice a week.

If this is you, Thinsulin provides a simple adjustment. Regardless of whether you're awake, or it's nighttime or daytime, your breakfast and dinner remain the same. In other words, if you work the night shift and you come into work at 7 p.m. and leave the hospital at 7 a.m., you would eat breakfast in the morning around 7 a.m. and dinner at about 5 p.m. before you go to work. So even when you shift back to your normal schedule of sleeping at night, your breakfast and dinner remain at the same time. However, the timing of your snacks and lunch will change. A good rule of thumb is to remember that the raw nuts as an afternoon snack will always occur when there's a long gap between two meals. If you're sleeping at night, that evening snack of raw nuts typically should occur between 4 and 5 p.m. However, if you work the night shift for twelve hours, your first break is around 8 p.m. At that time, eat one portion of a low-GI fruit. When it's your "lunchtime," usually around 11:30 p.m. or midnight, eat your lunch with green, leafy vegetables and meat. At around 3 to 4 a.m., you might feel tired and hungry. This is a good time to eat a handful of raw nuts to hold you through until breakfast. Make sure you eat some breakfast before you go to sleep in the morning.

Once you transition back to your normal day schedule, make sure that you're still eating breakfast, snack, lunch, snack, and dinner. You just shift the lunch back to your regular time (around noontime) and keep the low-GI fruit as a morning snack and a handful of nuts in the afternoon.

WHAT CAN I EAT FOR BREAKFAST?

It can be difficult to mix up your food choices for breakfast. It seems like there are many more choices for lunch and dinner. That's not entirely correct. Breakfast actually gives you an additional choice to eat dairy products such as plain yogurt and cheese in addition to your protein. If you're sick and tired of eating plain yogurt with fresh berries, consider freezing the berries along with the plain yogurt to make a new "shake" for breakfast. Once you've used up the low-GI fruits in the morning in your yogurt, then you can't eat another portion of fruits as your morning snack. Instead, consider eating celery or other vegetables instead of another fruit.

Boiling the egg whites the night before can save you some time the next morning. You can enjoy hard-boiled egg whites, but you might get tired of eating them after a while. Mix it up with another convenient breakfast choice, cheese. Yes, one portion of cheese. Any type of cheese for breakfast. You can even drink a juice for breakfast. Just make sure that your healthy juice doesn't contain potatoes, corn, carrots, or beets and more than one portion of low-GI fruits.

If you want bacon and egg whites, that's OK. Just don't eat this every day, especially if you have high cholesterol. You can have left-over lunch or dinner for breakfast. Some of our patients enjoy making a huge pot of soup that doesn't contain any foods that would spike their insulin level. The broth is made from chicken along with cabbage and other nonstarchy vegetables. You can use soy products or even hamburger patties to eat for breakfast.

Whatever you choose to eat, just know that there are a lot more foods that you haven't thought about. You just have to put on your

Thinsulin hat, be creative, and explore the different menus the world has to offer.

IS THINSULIN COMPATIBLE WITH CERTAIN MEDICAL CONDITIONS?

At our weight-loss office, we collect a thorough medical history for all our patients. Certain medical conditions preclude patients from taking certain pharmacotherapies. A good medical history will also help determine what adjustments, if any, are needed for them to be on the Thinsulin Program. It's important to get an annual physical examination with your primary care physician. Before you start any weight-loss program, it's always best to discuss its parameters with your physician first. Let's touch on a few important medical considerations as related to Thinsulin.

Type 2 diabetes. If you take medications for type 2 diabetes, you're at risk for hypoglycemia, or low blood glucose, when you cut out foods that lower the insulin level. Therefore, you need to be under medical supervision if you decide to do Thinsulin or any other weight-loss program. Some oral antidiabetic medications are more likely to cause hypoglycemia than others, but a dosage adjustment might be needed to minimize hypoglycemic episodes. We have patients with type 2 diabetes who have done very well on Thinsulin. Not only were they successful with losing weight, some were able to stop taking metformin, a medication used to treat diabetes, altogether. For those who require insulin injections, you'll need to be under close medical supervision if you go on a low-carb diet or on Thinsulin. You'll need to monitor your blood sugar when you wake up and before you sleep, and at breakfast, lunch, and dinner. Most likely, your physician might need to decrease your insulin dosage in order to minimize hypoglycemia.

For those with diabetes doing Thinsulin, continue to break down what you eat into five groups. Remember the traffic light analogy?

You definitely want to avoid sweets as a drink, dessert and snacks as well as starchy vegetables such as potatoes, corn, carrots, and beets. However, you don't have to be as strict on the grains if you have diabetes. To minimize the risks for hypoglycemia, it's recommended that you continue to eat one portion of healthy grains (brown rice, wheat bread, barley, quinoa, or oatmeal) twice a day, either at breakfast, lunch, or dinner. You would eat at least one portion of green, leafy vegetables along with protein. Your snacks would be the same of one fresh, low-GI fruit (apple, orange, grapes, or berries) in the morning and a portion of raw nuts in the evening. Patients with type 2 diabetes often have an elevated baseline insulin level. Therefore, if you cut back on foods that would spike insulin further, you'll still have a drop in insulin level if you're eating a healthy grain. At some point, you can consider cutting out healthy grains to help with the weight loss, but you must do this under close medical supervision. You can only consider that if you're able to reduce your antidiabetic medication dosage and have no hypoglycemic episodes.

Cardiac disease. If you have heart disease, high blood pressure, heart attacks, or strokes, it's important that you lose weight in order to reduce further risks of heart attacks and strokes. The difficult part is to know what to do. Due to your health you're unable to exercise, so you'll need to rely on changing the way that you eat in order to lose weight. Thinsulin is compatible with this population. If you're not taking any antidiabetic medications, you're not at risk for hypoglycemia. Therefore, you can follow the Thinsulin Program similar to what has been described in this book. The major exception is limiting your saturated fat intake. In other words, don't eat fried food. Try steaming, grilling or baking your meat and vegetables instead. You may have unsalted nuts as your afternoon snack.

Pregnancy. It's not recommended that you go on any weight-loss program while you're pregnant. You want to gain a healthy weight so that your fetus will have enough nutrients. Pregnancy is not a good time for you to lose weight. However, if you're packing on the pounds and are at risk for gestational diabetes, then you can apply the principles of Thinsulin to help get your blood sugar and weight under control. The adjustments are similar to a person with diabetes. A greater emphasis is placed on eating plenty of green, leafy vegetables and protein that won't spike insulin. You may have one portion of healthy grains per day. You absolutely need to avoid any sweets as a drink, dessert, or snack. If you're full, you're less likely to give in to the cravings.

Mental Illness. It's difficult to live with a mental illness. It's even more difficult to control the weight gain when the very same medication that's used to stabilize the mental illness contributes to weight gain. If you're taking medications that block serotonin 5HT2c receptors, you're going to feel hungry and not-full all the time, causing your body to crave and eat more. This is where pharmacotherapy for weight management might be helpful in countering the effects of antipsychotic medications and mood stabilizers. The Thinsulin Program takes a comprehensive approach that is beneficial in helping obese patients with mental illness lose weight and keep it off. It's important to feel full with your meals so that you're less likely to cheat on sweets and grains. Therefore, make sure to eat plenty of green, leafy vegetables first, and then at least one to two portions of protein at lunch and dinner.

Appendix A

MEDICATIONS FOR WEIGHT MANAGEMENT

Perception of obesity has changed over the years. In the past, obesity was considered simply a lifestyle problem induced by the environment. The view of obesity began to shift slowly in 2013, when the American Medical Association declared it to be a medical disease, with recognized symptoms and complex causes.

Our view of weight-loss medications, however, has been slower to change. Some expect these prescriptions to serve as panaceas that will allow them to drop loads of weight without lifting a finger. That's simply not the case. While some prescriptions can produce short-term weight loss, they aren't the smoking gun in the anti-obesity arsenal. You can't expect to lose real, lasting weight by popping any of these prescriptions without changing your eating habits.

Another school of thought believes these medications should never be used because it doesn't consider that you still have to change the way that you eat. If you're motivated enough, you'll have the willpower to walk away from the wrong foods and exercise more. While there's some truth to that, is it realistic? This thinking perpetuates the same old stigma and sets us back to the old, judgmental days where we view obesity as a result of personal weakness rather than as a disease.

We—Charles and Tu—consider ourselves to be disciplined people. We've got to be in order to manage our busy careers along with our personal lives as husbands, fathers, and friends. But if you ask these two Asian guys to give up rice and noodles, you'd better give us something good to help us walk away! It's not because we lack willpower, but the truth is, it's hard to break habits that we've developed over our lifetimes. And, since we have difficulty doing it ourselves, how can we expect our patients to?

For us, it's difficult to give up rice or noodles. For others, it might be bread, potatoes, corn, or tortillas. For you, it might be ice cream, chips, or other comfort foods. If you find it difficult to walk away from these foods on your own, don't worry. You're not alone. Billions of people struggle with this very same issue worldwide.

That's why the American Association of Clinical Endocrinologists (AACE), in 2013, came out with a treatment guideline that recommends starting pharmacotherapy (a.k.a., taking medications) along with lifestyle modifications as an initial treatment for obesity. Soon after, the National Heart, Lung, and Blood Institute (NHLBI), National Lipids Association (NLA), American Heart Association (AHA), American College of Cardiology (ACC), The Obesity Society (TOS), and the American Society of Bariatric Physicians (ASBP) published similar recommendations. For many people with a lifelong history of obesity, pharmacotherapy, including FDA-approved prescription medications like phentermine and the recently approved Qsymia®, Belviq®, Contrave™, and Saxenda®, can play an important role in helping them gain control of what they eat. If we look at smokers who want to quit, we see that they're often given a boost from Nicorette gum or prescribed medications such as Zyban® or Chantix® to reduce nicotine cravings in addition to smoking-cessation classes.

The medical community now refers to these medications as pharmacotherapies, rather than weight-loss medications. Are these terms basically saying the same thing? Not necessarily! "Weight-loss medications" imply that if you take these medications, you'll lose weight. But that's not accurate at all. If you take a prescription medication and eat exactly the same junk foods and drink sodas, don't be surprised if you don't lose weight. Pharmacotherapy is about weight management—targeting either the hunger or satiety and cravings might make it easier for you to resist doughnuts, sweets, and grains so that you're able to walk away from these indulgences. These medications interfere with the brain signals that make you feel full or not hungry. If you don't succumb to your cravings, you're able to lower your insulin level and eventually burn fat. The medications don't directly lower your insulin level, but help jump-start your weight-loss program by giving you more control over your appetite or satiety. These medications are only part of a treatment (therapy).

In our brick-and-mortar practice, we give our patients the option for pharmacotherapy to help them control their appetite or satiety. Whether or not our patients take medication, they lose the same amount of weight if they follow our program. That's because we teach Thinsulin to everyone. If patients follow the program correctly, they'll lose as much weight as those who are prescribed medications! As long as they lower their insulin level, their body will burn fat. It's as simple as that.

The decision to use pharmacotherapy is a personal choice. You know yourself best. Talk to your doctor about the new treatment options. However, understand that there's no such thing as a weight-loss pill. You still need to change your eating habits. Thinsulin will help you change your thinking and eating behavior, and can be used with or without pharmacotherapy.

REGULATION OF FOOD INTAKE

Before we talk about the different pharmacotherapy options, we want to help you understand how the brain regulates food intake. So, kick off your shoes and put your feet up! This will be a bit like a mini-refresher course in biology, and we think you'll be impressed by how much your brain does for you (free of charge—and without your even having to ask!).

Appetite and hunger are both sensations that represent a desire and a physiological need to eat, respectively. In contrast, satiety is the sensation of feeling full.

Different organs interact through a complex network of signals to maintain energy balance. An area of the brain called the hypothalamus regulates your body's food intake and energy expenditure (calories you burn). In particular, the arcuate nucleus of the hypothalamus is the key circuitry that regulates hunger and satiety. It receives signals from several hormones and peptides made by the gut and adipose tissue, such as insulin, leptin, ghrelin, and glucagon-like peptide-1 (GLP-1). In a fasting state, ghrelin and insulin stimulate the arcuate nucleus to cause hunger and increase appetite in order to make you eat.

On the other hand, hormones and peptides such as leptin and GLP-1 stimulate the arcuate nucleus to increase satiety or sensation of fullness. Hence, this makes you want to stop eating and increases resting energy expenditure. In addition, the neurons of the hypothalamus also release beta-endorphin, which acts to counter the reduction in food intake. The brain has this regulatory feedback loop to ensure that you don't go too long without eating. (Although if you're anything like us, you don't need a reminder to eat!)

Now, isn't the brain, well, smart? It's always looking out for you. It always has your back (and your legs, arms, feet, and every other body part). We know this is very detailed, but we want you to understand how your brain works. Now, let's put this into practice. Suppose you haven't eaten anything all morning. This causes your body to produce ghrelin. Ghrelin stimulates the arcuate nucleus to make you feel hungry.

Once you eat, your body has to know how much you can eat so that it can keep you from overeating. If you eat a lot of carbs or sweets, your pancreas produces insulin to promote lowering the blood sugar while telling the body to store fat. The fat cells produce leptin, and cells located in the lower gastrointestinal (GI) tract produce GLP-1. These hormones and peptides travel to the brain and stimulate the arcuate nucleus to increase satiety. As a result—bingo! You feel full so you stop eating. GLP-1 also inhibits glucagon release after meals.

(The pancreas releases glucagon into the bloodstream when glucose is too low.) That's why GLP-1 agonists such as Victoza® are FDA-approved for the management of type 2 diabetes as well as chronic weight management under the brand name Saxenda®.

Another mechanism that communicates with your brain to tell you that you're full involves the mu-opioid receptors (MORs) located in the walls of the portal vein, a major blood vessel that drains blood from the gut. The type of food you eat can affect your sensation of fullness.

When you stimulate the MORs in the portal vein, this communicates with the hypothalamus to tell you to eat more. On the other hand, when you block the MORs, the opposite occurs. Your hypothalamus tells you you're full, so that you'll stop eating.

In a study published in *Cell*, a peer-reviewed scientific journal, researchers reported that the products of digested proteins, or peptides, can *block* the MORs. Therefore, high-protein foods such as lean meat will make you feel full. That's also the reason why you should snack on raw nuts in the afternoon—the high-protein nuts will block the MORs in the wall linings of the portal veins to increase satiety. As a result, you're less likely to cheat before dinner.

Next, we'll spend some time talking about the different pharmacotherapy options currently available. These sections are meant to provide you with some background rather than to give you any form of medical advice. Talk to your doctor to weigh the risks and benefits, and consider all possible alternative treatments before you take any prescription medications.

Pharmacotherapies target different mechanisms in the body to manage obesity. They may interfere with nutrient absorption, suppress appetite, increase satiety, or affect brain signaling.

MEDICATIONS THAT INTERFERE WITH NUTRIENT ABSORPTION

Orlistat, marketed as Xenical®, or its over-the-counter version, Alli®, was approved by the FDA in 1999 as a long-term treatment for obesity management in conjunction with a reduced-calorie diet. Orlistat works by blocking the pancreatic enzyme lipase that normally breaks down dietary fat in the gastrointestinal tract. Orlistat has been shown in a four-year clinical trial involving 3,304 overweight patients to have a mean weight loss of more than 11 percent, compared with a six percent mean weight loss with a placebo. Because of its mechanism of action, Orlistat can prevent absorption of fat-soluble vitamins such as vitamin A, D, E, and K, leading to a small but significant decrease in vitamin levels. Therefore, it's recommended to take a multivitamin daily if you're taking Orlistat. In addition, because it prevents fat absorption, the side effects of Orlistat can be uncomfortable and embarrassing. In the clinical studies, common gastrointestinal symptoms of fatty, oily stool, increased bowel movements, and flatus (gas), have been reported, leading to potential risk of oily spotting.

MEDICATIONS THAT SUPPRESS APPETITE

In the late 1800s, thyroid extract was used as an early remedy for obesity, but it resulted in hyperthyroidism and other serious side effects. The drug dinitrophenyl was used in the 1930s to reduce weight by speeding up metabolism, but it resulted in cataracts, nerve malfunction, and even death from hypothermia. The drug can still be bought on the Internet today, and is sometimes misused by extreme dieters or bodybuilders looking to diminish every bit of body fat.

At one point in the 1940s, amphetamines were used as an antiobesity drug, but their addictive properties kept them off the shelves. Phenmetrazine (Preludin®), a central nervous system stimulant of the morpholine chemical class, was approved by the FDA in 1956, but has since been withdrawn from the market due to concerns of abuse and addiction. In 1959, three drugs that are chemically and pharmacologically related to amphetamines were approved by the FDA for short-term use in the management of obesity: phentermine (Adipex-P®, Ionamin®, Suprenza®), phendimetrazine tartrate (Adipost®, Anorex-SR®, Appecon®, Bontril PDM®, Bontril SR®,

Melfiat®, Obezine®, Phendiet®, Plegine®, Prelu-2®, and Statobex®), and diethylpropion (Tenuate®, Tenuate Dospan®, Tepanil®).

Phentermine, a norepinephrine reuptake inhibitor, is thought to promote weight loss by activating the sympathetic nervous system, with a resulting decrease in food intake and increase in resting energy expenditure, or the number of calories you would burn if you rested all day. Studies show that 60 percent of patients taking phentermine lose between 5 to 15 percent of body weight in three months, which is significantly more than those who received only lifestyle counseling. Phentermine is the most commonly prescribed appetite suppressant, accounting for 50 percent of all prescriptions. Side effects include dry mouth, insomnia, constipation, and high blood pressure. The medication, which is similar to amphetamines, is also potentially addictive. Phentermine should be avoided in people with moderate to severe high blood pressure, cardiovascular disease, hyperthyroidism, substance abuse, and anxiety disorders, during pregnancy and while breast-feeding.

All stimulants, including weight-loss supplements, are believed to increase heart rate and blood pressure, making it dangerous for people with cardiovascular disease to use them. Weight-loss supplements, such as ephedra (which the FDA banned in 2004), ephedrine, and caffeine work by suppressing the appetite, but manufacturers of these supplements often make unsubstantiated claims that aren't supported by long-term scientific evidence or safety data. Be wary of anything that promotes a "miracle cure" in weight loss. Although green tea beverage consumption (four cups per day) or extract supplementation (two capsules per day) have been shown to decrease body weight and BMI, it's simply incorrect to announce miraculous claims from those small studies. Such great misunderstanding on the subject ensued that on January 26, 2015, the Federal Trade Commission (FTC) banned the promotion of green coffee bean supplements on TV programs. The supplement manufacturer had been advertising all over, claiming that people taking the green coffee beans would lose 17 pounds in twelve weeks, even without diet restriction or exercise.

MEDICATIONS THAT INCREASE SATIETY

It's believed that the neurotransmitter serotonin 5-HT system plays a role in controlling satiety. Studies show that stimulation of receptors in the hypothalamus called $5HT_{2C}$ receptors affects satiety. Dr. Laurence Tecott, MD, PhD, a scientist at the University of California, San Francisco, bred a strain of rats that had no functional $5HT_{2C}$ receptors. He observed that the rats ate more and became obese.

Fenfluramine (Pondimin®) is thought to work as an appetite suppressant through the stimulation of $5HT_{2C}$ receptors. The FDA approved fenfluramine in 1972, and its active compound, dexfenfluramine (Redux®), in 1995, for the short-term management of obesity. A landmark study completed in 1992 showed that fenfluramine, used in combination with the weight-loss drug phentermine, otherwise known as "fen-phen," was very effective for short-term (generally three months) weight loss. The FDA never approved the use of these drugs together, but it surged in popularity as many doctors prescribed the combination off-label for weight loss. In 1997, a study in the *New England Journal of Medicine* from the Mayo Clinic reported a possible correlation between heart valve damage and the use of "fen-phen." Subsequently, another independent study showed that patients using the "fen-phen" combination for longer than three months were twenty-three times more likely to develop primary pulmonary hypertension, a serious, permanent lung condition that can lead to breathing problems, heart failure, and death. In September 1997, the FDA requested the removal of fenfluramine and dexfenfluramine from the market. For the next few years, many researchers debated the cause of pulmonary hypertension and heart valve damage. In December 2000, Dr. R.B. Rothman published studies showing that fenfluramine and dexfenfluramine's stimulation of 5HT2B receptors was the likely cause of the heart valve damage. Phentermine, on the other hand, doesn't affect the serotonin system or 5HT2B receptors, or cause valvular heart disease. Phentermine is still considered safe for short-term use.

Sibutramine (Meridia®) was approved by the FDA in 1997 for the management of obesity, including weight loss and the maintenance of weight loss, in conjunction with a reduced-calorie diet. Sibutramine is a neurotransmitter reuptake inhibitor that ultimately increases the serotonin, norepinephrine, and dopamine levels in the brain, thereby enhancing satiety and reducing appetite. Unfortunately, a large, randomized, controlled study, "Sibutramine Cardiovascular Outcomes (SCOUT)," of more than ten thousand patients showed that a higher number of cardiovascular events, such as heart attacks and strokes, occurred with patients taking sibutramine compared with those taking placebos. Sibutramine was eventually withdrawn from the market in October 2010.

Given the precarious history associated with these weight-loss medications, it took nearly thirteen years for the FDA to grant another pharmacotherapy option for obesity. Lorcaserin (Belviq®), developed by Arena Pharmaceuticals and marketed by Eisai Inc., was approved by the FDA on June 27, 2012 as an adjunct to a reduced-calorie diet and increased physical activity for chronic weight management in adults with an initial BMI of 30 or greater, or 27 or greater in the presence of at least one weight-related condition such as high blood pressure, high cholesterol, or type 2 diabetes. Common side effects include constipation, dizziness, dry mouth, fatigue, headache, and nausea. Belviq® might cause certain serious side effects such as serotonin syndrome if taken with drugs that increase serotonin levels. It shouldn't be taken while pregnant.

Belviq® is thought to work by selectively stimulating serotonin 2C ($5HT_{2C}$) receptors while not stimulating serotonin 2B (5HT2B) receptors, at clinically effective doses. The minimal stimulation of 5HT2B receptors reduces the risk for heart valve problems. The mechanism of action for weight loss is similar to fenfluramine, except it doesn't have the risks for heart valve or pulmonary hypertension problems due to its lack of 5HT2B receptors' stimulation.

Two Phase III trials of Belviq® showed that those taking the medication lost between 4 to 6 percent of body weight in one year. Those who completed the study lost a bit more, showing an average loss of 8 percent of body weight in a year. There was no increase in numbers of valvulopathy, or heart valve damage.

A third study, the Bloom DM study, indicated that patients with type 2 diabetes mellitus taking Belviq® compared with those taking a sugar pill, or placebo, had a 27 point drop in the fasting blood sugar level (compared with an 11.9 point drop on placebo), and an impressive 0.9 point drop in the hemoglobin A1C level (compared with a 0.4 point drop on placebo) after one year. Hemoglobin A1C measures the three-month average of the blood sugar levels, so it's a better indicator of the long-term improvement.

What's impressive about Belviq® is the fact that it has no known mechanism to treat diabetes, and yet, these improvements are comparable with many of the diabetes pills that we currently use. Belviq® is thought to produce weight loss due to its stimulation of the serotonin 2C ($5HT_{2C}$) receptors in the hypothalamus, but how would it produce such a significant improvement in blood sugar in patients with type 2 diabetes? We don't have an answer, but we suspect that Belviq® might make it easier for patients to comply with their American Diabetic Association (ADA) diet consisting of low carbs and high protein. In other words, if you're trying to lower your insulin level by eating fewer carbs and more protein, Belviq® might make it easier for you to follow through by staying away from carbs and sweets.

On December 23, 2014, the FDA approved its fourth drug for chronic weight management since 2012. Saxenda® is approved for people with a BMI over 30, or a BMI of 27 with weight-related conditions such as high blood pressure, high cholesterol, or type 2 diabetes, along with a reduced-calorie diet and exercise. Saxenda® works by mimicking the activities of the natural peptide GLP-1 so it has to be injected as a medication rather than taken as a pill by mouth.

Three clinical trials involving more than forty-eight hundred obese and overweight patients showed an average weight loss of 4.5 percent or 10.5 pounds weight loss from baseline compared with placebo after twelve months. Sixty-two percent treated with Saxenda® lost at least 5 percent of their body weight compared with 34 percent treated with placebo. The most common side effects are constipation, diarrhea, low blood sugar, nausea, and vomiting. Saxenda® should not be used in patients with a personal or family history of medullary thyroid cancer.

Combination Medications Affecting Appetite and/or Satiety

Qsymia®, manufactured and marketed by Vivus Inc., was approved by the FDA on July 17, 2012, as an adjunct to a reduced-calorie diet and increased physical activity for chronic weight management in adults with a BMI of 30 or greater, or 27 or greater in the presence of at least one weight-related condition such as high blood pressure, high cholesterol, or type 2 diabetes. Qsymia® combines two available generic medications: phentermine, an appetite suppressant, with topiramate, a drug approved for epileptic seizures and migraine headaches. While phentermine is thought to suppress appetite, topiramate is thought to increase satiety, or feeling full. High-dose Qsymia®, consisting of 15 mg of phentermine and 92 mg of topiramate, helps patients lose between 6.7 percent to 8.9 percent over placebo.

Qsymia® is not for patients with hyperthyroidism, glaucoma, during or within fourteen days following the administration of monoamine oxidase inhibitors, and during pregnancy. Qsymia® can cause an increase in heart rate and cognitive dulling. It can also cause fetal harm due to the topiramate component. Therefore, you must do a pregnancy test prior to starting Qsymia®. Side effects include altered taste sensation, constipation, dizziness, dry mouth, insomnia, and tingling of hands and feet.

Another medication, Contrave™, developed by Orexigen Therapeutics, Inc., and marketed by Takeda Pharmaceutical Company Limited, was approved by the FDA on September 10, 2014, as a treatment option for chronic weight management in addition to a reduced-calorie diet and physical activity. The drug is approved for use in adults with a BMI of 30 or greater or adults with a BMI of 27 or greater who have at least one weight-related condition such as high blood pressure, high cholesterol, or type 2 diabetes.

Contrave™ is a combination of two drugs already on the market: naltrexone, which is approved for opioid addiction (1984) and alcohol dependence (1995), marketed as ReVia®, and bupropion, marketed as Wellbutrin® as an antidepressant (1985), and as Zyban® for smoking cessation (1997). By itself, the medication causes minimal weight loss by affecting the hypothalamus to promote satiety and reduced eating. But the combination of both naltrexone and bupropion seems to yield a more potent, sustained effect on food intake than either medication alone, although no one truly understands how the combination works for weight loss.

In addition, the combination of both medications might regulate the brain's mesolimbic reward pathways, leading to a reduction in reward values and goal-oriented behaviors.

Multiple clinical trials studying the effectiveness of Contrave™ involved approximately forty-five hundred obese and overweight patients with and without significant weight-related conditions in treatment for one year. All patients received lifestyle modification that consisted of a reduced-calorie diet and regular physical activity.

On average, patients taking Contrave™ lose 5 to 10 percent of their starting weight, with the average weight loss of 13.4 pounds. In a fifty-six-week study looking at Contrave™ combined with intensive lifestyle modification counseling, those taking Contrave™ lost about 9 percent of their starting weight compared with those on placebo who lost just 5 percent. So, if a person's starting weight is 220 pounds, this person would lose about 20 pounds after one year of treatment with Contrave™, while the person taking a placebo would end up losing roughly 11 pounds.

Contrave™ shouldn't be taken by patients with a seizure disorder, eating disorder, who are pregnant or planning to get pregnant, or who have acute hepatitis or liver failure. Potential seizures and liver damage might occur in higher dosages, so it's recommended to stay within the recommended dose of naltrexone (8 mg.) and buproprion (360 mg.) per day taken in a divided dose. Like in other antidepressants, taking Contrave™ carries an increased risk of suicidal thoughts and behaviors; serious neuropsychiatric events have occurred in patients taking bupropion.

MEDICATIONS THAT AFFECT BRAIN SIGNALING

While weight-loss medications mimic natural peptides or bind to brain receptors, an implantable device was recently approved by the FDA to change the food signaling between the stomach and brain.

On January 14, 2015, the FDA approved an implantable device called the Maestro® Rechargeable System, the first-ever weight-loss device involved in the workings of the nerve pathway between the stomach and brain that controls hunger and satiety. Although this isn't a medication, it's a device made by EnteroMedics that's implanted in the abdomen, with wires attached to the vagus nerve in-between the esophagus and stomach. By sending electrical pulses to the vagus nerve every several minutes, the Maestro® System tricks the brain into feeling full.

The vagus nerve stretches from the brain all the way down to the stomach to control several important activities: 1) When to expand to fit more food; 2) When to secrete chemicals to break down food; and 3) When to contract to process the food. In addition, when the stomach stretches after you eat, this activates the stretch receptors that send signals along the vagus nerve on a different pathway to the hypothalamus to increase satiety, so that you can stop eating.

In a clinical trial that included 233 patients with a BMI greater than 35, more than half of the patients who received the Maestro® System lost at least 20 percent of the excess weight, and 38 percent of them lost at least 25 percent of the excess weight after a year of treatment. Those who didn't receive the device still lost weight. In fact, nearly one-third lost at least 20 percent and more than one-fifth lost at least 25 percent of their excess weight.

Not all adults are eligible for the devices. Only adults who haven't been able to lose the weight in five years with a weight-loss program and who have a BMI over 35 with at least one other obesity-related condition (such as type 2 diabetes) may be eligible for the device. Serious adverse events include pain, nausea, vomiting, and surgical complications.

The Maestro® System offers patients a chance to lose weight without having to change the way that they eat with the device. They can simply turn it on when they want to feel full and turn it off when they no longer need it. However, we don't think it's going to be that simple. Having the device may help, but we still believe that you'll need to change your way of thinking through psychotherapy if you want to lose weight and keep it off.

BREAKING THE OBESITY CYCLE

Obesity is commonly seen as a consequence of unhealthy eating and lack of physical activity. From that standpoint, it's easy to blame a person for being obese because they lack willpower or have a character flaw. But this view of obesity has shifted, and the medical community now recognizes that it's a chronic disease due to genetic, biological, behavioral, and psychological factors.

Job, family, and relationship stressors often lead to depression. Studies suggest a strong relationship between obesity and depression, especially among women. Depression can lead to poor food choices and decreased physical activity, resulting in weight gain. As weight increases, this can cause problems with self-confidence and body image, which, in turn, can lead to eating disorders, major depression, and further weight gain. It's a vicious cycle!

You can break this cycle by moving away from a diet mentality to one that envisions weight loss as a journey. In your journey, pharmacotherapies might be an option to give you a better chance of walking away from certain foods without thinking of them all day. Pharmacotherapies work by blocking absorption of nutrients, suppressing appetite, increasing satiety or feeling full, or affecting brain signaling.

Physicians now have more medications in their arsenal to treat obesity, but the concept of weight loss by lowering your insulin level remains unchanged. You simply can't change your biology. Whether or not you decide to pursue pharmacotherapy as an option, keep in mind that you still have to learn how to change your way of thinking if you want to lose weight and keep it off. Thinsulin will help you achieve your goals no matter what you decide.

Appendix B

WEIGHT-LOSS SURGERY AND THINSULIN

Weight-loss surgery is very effective in helping you to lose weight, but not everyone can afford or qualify for surgery. Even if you're able to get bariatric surgery, ask yourself if you're ready to make the required lifestyle commitment. Surgery will not magically lead to weight loss without effort. You still have to develop new eating and exercise habits. You still have to work hard to fight the food cravings. Ultimately, you still have to commit to a new lifestyle. That's why the Thinsulin Program may offer a solution to help you, even if you're contemplating bariatric surgery or have already had surgery.

If you lose weight with the Thinsulin Program, you may increase your chance to qualify for surgery—or better yet, you may not *need* surgery. If you've already had the weight-loss procedure, the Thinsulin Program will allow you to stay on track by helping you to change your way of thinking and modify your eating habits. You'll develop new skills and tools to keep losing weight and prevent weight regain.

In this section, we'll take a look at the different types of weight-loss surgeries available so that you can consider with your physician whether one may be right for you.

BARIATRIC SURGERY

The word "bariatric" is derived from the Greek words "baros," which means "weight," and "iatrikos," which means "medicine." The first bariatric surgery performed in humans, the jejunoileal bypass, was reported in 1954. Because the procedure bypasses the small intestine, patients were unable to digest and absorb nutrients, leading to severe protein and micronutrient deficiencies. As a result, most surgeons abandoned this method in the late 1970s.

But bariatric weight-loss surgeries have come a long way since then, and according to the Centers for Disease Control and Prevention (CDC), weight-loss surgery is gaining popularity. From 1996 to 2007, the annual rate of weight-loss surgery increased from 3.3 per hundred thousand American adults to 22.4 per hundred thousand. To qualify for surgery, a person must have a BMI of at least 40 or more, or 35 or more if they have an obesity-associated condition such as sleep apnea or type 2 diabetes.

Many experts consider bariatric surgery to be the most effective treatment for obesity, helping to improve obesity-related conditions and long-term weight maintenance. Researchers analyzed data from eleven randomized, controlled trials involving 796 obese adults with a BMI between 30 and 52 to see the effectiveness of bariatric surgery compared with nonsurgical methods such as behavioral therapy, dietary changes, increased physical activity, and the use of pharmacotherapy, over a two-year period. The study reported that patients who had bariatric surgery lost more body weight (an average of 57.2 pounds) and had higher remission rates of type 2 diabetes and metabolic syndrome, compared with those who followed nonsurgical methods.

Today, most bariatric surgery is conducted by laparoscopic surgery, a minimally-invasive procedure that requires only a few small incisions about half an inch in size. These tiny incisions lead to less scarring, a shorter hospital stay, and fewer potential complications. Although it's obvious why most people would prefer this type of surgery, not all patients qualify. Only those who have complex medical problems, are extremely obese, or have had previous stomach surgery qualify. All invasive surgical procedures carry potential risks of complications, including bleeding, infection, blockage or tears in the bowels, and even a need for further surgery. For either procedure, you may experience pain at the site of incisions. Therefore, you may need pain meds for a few weeks.

Although the exact mechanism of weight loss is complex, it is thought that bariatric surgery leads to weight loss by these three mechanisms:

1. Restriction: reduces the size of the stomach to limit the amount of food intake
2. Malabsorption: limits the absorption of foods in the intestine
3. Combination of restriction and malabsorption

Restriction

The **LAP-BAND® System** is a popular, relatively simple surgery in which an adjustable silicone band is implanted around the opening to the stomach to help you feel full and lose weight. The procedure, which takes less than one hour, is usually done laparoscopically on an outpatient basis. The versatile band can be tightened, loosened, or even removed if there are complications. It won't work at all, however, if you don't change your eating habits. For example, if you enjoy ice cream and sodas on a regular basis, the band, no matter how tight, won't help you to feel full. You'll still need to eat foods that don't raise insulin in order to lose weight. If you follow the band protocol correctly, weight loss ranges from 45 to 75 percent after two years. A study published in *Obesity* showed a mean weight loss of 65 percent after one year with significant improvement in lipid problems, high blood pressure, and diabetes.

A second bariatric surgery that works by limiting the amount of food intake is the **gastric sleeve**, also known as sleeve gastrectomy. This one-hour laparoscopic procedure reshapes the size of the stomach into a narrow tube. After surgery, the stomach is much smaller (about the size of a banana), allowing you to feel full after eating less food. The gastric sleeve has a good success rate: people lose an average of 33 percent of their excess body weight in the first year. For a person who is 120 pounds overweight, this would mean losing about 40 pounds in the first year. Remember, it's important to eat right for success and to follow a low insulin diet after surgery. Unlike the LAP-BAND®, the gastric sleeve isn't reversible, so consider all the risks and talk to your doctor before making the decision to undergo this surgery.

Malabsorption

A less common bariatric surgery that works by limiting absorption of foods is called **biliopancreatic diversion (BPD)**. It's a complex, high-risk surgery that is used as a last resort for someone who is extremely obese (a BMI of 50 or a BMI of 40, with significant health problems like heart disease, high cholesterol, type 2 diabetes, and others). The surgery has several features. First, the lower stomach is removed. Second, the remaining upper stomach is connected directly to the jejunum, the middle part of the small intestine. Most foods are absorbed in the first part of the small intestine, called the duodenum. As a result of the surgery, the digested foods completely bypass the duodenum, leading to malabsorption, or weight loss. Although this procedure will lead to significant weight loss by not absorbing foods, you won't be absorbing important nutrients either, such as fat-soluble vitamins (vitamins A, D, E, and K) as well as iron, calcium, and vitamin B12. You'll need to take these supplements for the rest of your life or lack of these important nutrients may lead to anemia and osteoporosis.

A major side effect of this procedure is called "dumping syndrome." Now that the distance between the stomach and small intestines has been shortened, food can pass too quickly for many patients. This is characterized by nausea, diarrhea, weakness, light-headedness, fainting, fast heartbeat, and/or heart palpitations.

A variation of the BPD called the **BPD-DS,** or the duodenal switch, is designed to prevent the "dumping syndrome" by retaining a part of the stomach valve to control the release of food into the small intestine. The duodenum is also retained to minimize malabsorption.

According to the American Society of Metabolic and Bariatric Surgery, these two methods are the most successful of all bariatric surgeries. Many people lose at least 60 to 70 percent of their weight after five years. A study published in *World Journal of Surgery* reported that a series of 2,241 patients operated on with these procedures over a twenty-one-year period lost a mean 75 percent of their initial weight permanently. Eventually, people can resume eating at near normal food levels.

The downsides, however, are severe. These types of surgery hold greater rates of complications and risk of mortality than the other surgeries. As mentioned before, these surgeries can result in life-threatening nutritional deficiencies if not watched closely. As always, speak to your doctor before making the decision to undergo any bariatric surgery and consider them only as a last resort.

COMBINATION OF RESTRICTION AND MALABSORPTION

Gastric Bypass surgery—also known as Roux-en-Y gastric bypass—is the most widely performed surgery worldwide. The surgeon works two to four hours in an outpatient setting to create a small stomach pouch by dividing the stomach and attaching it to the small intestine. Weight loss will occur because the smaller stomach will hold less food (restriction). You will feel full after eating a small amount of food and liquid. The food bypasses the stomach and small intestine; the body will absorb fewer calories (malabsorption). People undergoing a gastric bypass lose an average of 50 to 75 percent of their excess weight after two years. On the downside, you may expect to see malabsorption issues, vitamin and mineral deficiencies, specifically vitamin B12, calcium, iron, and folate, as well as "dumping syndrome" with this procedure.

CANDIDATES FOR WEIGHT-LOSS SURGERY

To lose weight and avoid complications, you'll need to follow closely the diet and exercise program your doctor gives you. By losing this weight, you'll feel better, and many medical problems such as asthma, high blood pressure, high cholesterol, sleep apnea, and type 2 diabetes will improve or disappear altogether. The decision to undergo this surgery is not, however, to be taken lightly.

Is bariatric surgery right for you? Talk to your doctor first and weigh the risks and benefits of surgery. Do your due diligence. At the end, it comes down to your personal choice. Take into consideration some of these factors.

One consideration is the cost of bariatric surgery. The average cost is estimated to be $20,000 to $25,000, but it can vary widely by state. Check with your medical insurance to see if you're covered for this procedure.

Even if you can afford bariatric surgery, you will still have to undergo a comprehensive, multidisciplinary team assessment involving a psychological, medical, and nutritional evaluation before you are considered for bariatric surgery. A psychologist or psychiatrist will determine if you're psychologically fit for bariatric surgery. If you have poor adaptation skills, active depression, and other severe mental disorders, you may have poorer outcomes. A surgeon will determine if you're physically fit for surgery. Finally, a dietician will evaluate if you're able to comply with the new way of eating necessary for a successful outcome. If you're unable to follow through with postoperative care, you may not be a candidate for bariatric surgery due to a high failure rate.

Patients with the best outcomes after weight-loss surgery most commonly demonstrate active lifestyle changes with improved eating patterns and physical activity. In a study done by Dr. Rachel Goldman, she reported that more successful bariatric surgery patients had great activation in the part of the brain that is associated with self-control. In other words, the patients who were able to fight food cravings tended to have better outcomes and lost more weight.

LIPOSUCTION

Liposuction is not an alternative to weight loss. It's a plastic surgery intended for people who have one stubborn area of fat that won't budge with diet and exercise. It has become the most popular plastic surgery in America, surpassing breast augmentation surgery, with more than 363,000 operations a year. Liposuction removes fat from your body using suction. There are several techniques used to perform liposuction. The most traditional form, suction-assisted liposuction (SAL), draws fat out from a vacuum via small cuts made in the skin. A newer liposuction technique, laser-assisted liposuction (LAL), such as Smartlipo and Slimlipo™, use lasers to disrupt the fat cells and make fat removal less traumatic for the body.

Some people use liposuction as a way to control fat. They're often drawn to the before-and-after photos that show how quickly fat vanished after this cosmetic procedure. But are these results permanent? Absolutely not!

A new study published in the journal *Obesity* showed that the fat came back within one year, but not in the area where the fat was removed. It returned in different places. In the study conducted by Dr. Robert Eckel and his colleagues, nonobese women who had liposuction on their hips, thighs, and lower abdomen reported that the fat returned in the upper abdomen and triceps. However, most women in the study were still satisfied with the results even though the fat redistributed itself elsewhere.

Because liposuction isn't a substitute for a healthy lifestyle, liposuction shouldn't be considered as a weight-loss option. You may get instant results with thinner thighs or a flatter belly, but expect the fat to come back to different parts of the body if you don't change the way you eat. If you're able to naturally control your insulin levels to burn fat, you'll have a better chance of burning off the fat effectively to achieve lasting results. Even if you're able to remove fat, liposuction won't address the excess, loose skin caused by the rapid weight loss.

BODY CONTOURING

While it's a quick high to shed a lot of weight quickly, you'll soon discover that it's very hard to get rid of all the excess, hanging skin. For the readers who've gone through pregnancy, do you remember all the loose skin on your belly after childbirth? That's because your skin had been stretched to the max and lost its natural elasticity. Many people who have successfully lost a lot of weight (usually over 100 pounds) from bariatric surgery will see layers of sagging skin replacing layers of fat all over the body. When they look in the mirror, they will see a constant reminder of their past, even though they know that they're much healthier now.

Whether you've lost large amounts of weight through nonsurgical or surgical ways, body contouring plastic surgery removes excess, sagging skin so that you end up with a more normal appearance. You want to wait at least one year after bariatric surgery, when your weight stabilizes, before considering body contouring surgery.

A common plastic surgery that has been around for many years is the **tummy tuck**, also known as abdominoplasty. This surgery removes excess, loose skin along with fat. In most cases, it restores weakened muscles that may be caused by age, weight changes, or pregnancy. The end result is a smoother, firmer, and flatter abdomen. Remember, a tummy tuck is not a substitute for exercise or weight loss.

Body contouring surgery is different from tummy tuck surgery because excess skin is removed from multiple areas of the body. The most popular procedure is the lower body lift, where surgeons operate an average of six hours to remove excess skin from the abdomen, back, and outer thighs.

For upper body surgery, you need to wait about two months to give your body time to heal. You may choose a procedure called a **brachioplasty**, which removes sagging skin from your upper arms.

With any surgeries, you need at least two weeks of bed rest and up to six weeks of recovery time. There's also risk of infection, bleeding, blood clots, and scarring.

Body contouring surgery doesn't come cheap. The cost of the procedure varies based on the plastic surgeon's experiences. The average prices for a brachioplasty, tummy tuck, and lower body lift are $3700, $5,000, and $8,100 respectively. Most health insurance plans don't pay for this type of surgery.

—————

Surgery is a personal choice. The truth is, you know yourself best. Bariatric surgery has proven to be very effective for weight loss, but you still need to commit to a lifestyle change. The Thinsulin Program will help complement bariatric surgery so that you'll learn new skills to keep the weight off. If you've lost weight but still have some stubborn fat that you can't get rid of, liposuction might be an option, but be aware that the fat could come back without lifestyle changes. After significant weight loss, you might feel you want to consider body contouring surgery to remove excess, loose skin. If you choose surgery or not, just know that you still need a program to help you change your thinking and, ultimately, your habits. Thinsulin can get you there.

Acknowledgments

The authors would like to express sincere thanks to the folks at Perseus Books Group, specifically Renee Sedliar, for believing in this book. A big thank you to Renee and Kathryn McHugh for their close reading of this manuscript, and to Marco Pavia for his detailed watch over its design. We can't thank Dr. Daniel Amen enough for generously writing the foreword. The razor-sharp team of Sharon Bially and BookSavvy Public Relations worked tirelessly to get the word out on our behalf; Victor Abalos graciously contributed his inestimable expertise to champion this book. Thank you to our fabulous agent, Claire Gerus, for landing us the perfect publisher. Last, a special thank you to the Lorphen Medical patients who have graciously shared their stories and photos in this book.

Charles T. Nguyen, MD: I want to acknowledge and thank all my patients—you have served as my inspiration to write this book. Thanks to my talented friends, Hop Pham and Hoang Huynh, for the illustrations. I want to thank my parents for inspiring my brother and me to write. I want to thank my parents-in-law, Vinh and Dana Truong, for their support. I want to thank my brothers-in-law, Sam Truong, MD, and Peter Truong, DDS, and sister-in-law, Vangie Tran, FNP-BC, for their input. I want to thank Dr. Daniel Amen for his mentorship. Thanks to my good friend, Rick Ishitani, for introducing me to Mary Ann. This book would not have been possible if not for the editorial leadership and constant encouragement of Mary Ann Marshall. Through all of its ups and downs, thank you, Mary Ann, for being there for this amazing journey. Last, I want to thank my older brother, Tu Song-Anh Nguyen, MD, for sharing with me the role insulin plays in weight loss. Without him, this program would not have existed.

Tu Song-Anh Nguyen, MD: I would like to take this opportunity to thank my parents, Thuan Song Nguyen and Loan Ngoc Le, for their support, sacrifice, and guidance to help me to become who I am today. I sincerely want to thank my wife, Darlene Uyen Nguyen, for her encouragement and support in my journey through life. I want to thank my children, Koby and Ben, for the inspiration, joy and meaning they bring to my life. I also want to thank my brother and sisters. I especially want to thank Charles T. Nguyen, MD, who is not only my younger brother but truly my best friend and business partner, and his wife, Quynh-Tram Truong, DDS. I want to thank both of my younger sisters and their husbands: Diane Nguyen, MD, and Bao Trinh, PhD; and Irene Nguyen, PharmD, and Loi Tran, DO. I also want to thank Danny Tran, whose talents in IT helped to design our book website: www.thinsulinprogram.com. Furthermore, I want to thank my relatives, friends, and patients for inspiring me with the ideas to create the concepts in this book.

Mary Ann Marshall: I want to thank my parents, Allen and Ruth Marshall, for their never-ending support and good humor during the writing of this book. Thank you to the people who inspire me every day: Dr. Carolyn Johnston, Diane Paylor, Melissa Mackinnon, John McNeilly, Jeff Thomas, Alex Press, Pamela Rafalow Grossman, Andrea Todd, and the late Bill Dickman. A sincere thank you to Charles T. Nguyen, MD, for the pleasure and honor of working together. You are truly a brilliant thinker and we want to hear much more from you. Finally, I dedicate this book to my grandmother, Lucille Marshall.

REFERENCES

AACE Position Statement. *Endocr Prac.* 2012; 18 (5): 642–648.

Abenhaim L, Moride Y, Brenot F, Rich S, Benichou J, Kurz X, Higenbottam T, Oakley C, Wouters E, Aubier M, Simonneau G, Begaud B. "Appetite-suppressant drugs and the risk of primary pulmonary hypertension." *New Engl Journal Med. Aug.* 1996; 335 (9): 609–16.

Appelhans BM, Whited MC, Schneider KL, Pagoto SL. "Time to Abandon the Notion of Personal Choice in Dietary Counseling for Obesity?" *Journal Amer Diet Ass.* 2011; 111 (8): 1130–1136.

Appelhans BM, Whited MC, Schneider KL, Pagoto SL. "Time to Abandon the Notion of Personal Choice in Dietary Counseling for Obesity?" *Journal Amer Diet Ass.* 2011; 111 (8): 1130–1136.

Aronne LJ, Nelinson DS, Lillo JL. "Obesity as a disease state: a new paradigm for diagnosis and treatment." *Clinical Cornerstone.* 2009; 9 (4): 9–29.

Avena NM, Rada P, Hoebel BG. "Sugar and fat bingeing have notable differences in addictive-like behavior." *Journal Nutr.* Mar. 2009; 139 (3): 623–8.

Baker RC, Kirschenbaum DS. "Self-monitoring might be necessary for successful weight control." *Behav Ther.* 1993; 24: 377–94.

Basaranoglu M, Basaranoglu G, Sabuncu T, Sentürk H. "Fructose as a key player in the development of fatty liver disease." *World Journal Gastroenterol.* 2013; 19 (8): 1166–72.

Basu A, Sanchez K, Leyva MJ, Wu M, Betts NM, Aston CE, Lyons TJ. "Green Tea Supplementation Affects Body Weight, Lipids, and Lipid Peroxidation in Obese Subjects with Metabolic Syndrome." *Journal Am Coll Nutr.* Feb. 2010; 29 (1): 31–40.

Befort CA, Nollen N, Ellerbeck EF, Sullivan DK, Thomas JL, Ahluwalia JS. "Motivational interviewing fails to improve outcomes of a behavioral weight loss program for obese African American women: a pilot randomized trial." *Journal Behav Med.* 2008; 31: 367–377.

Bellisle F, Drewnowski A. "Intense sweeteners, energy intake and the control of body weight." *Eur J Clin Nutr.* 2007; 61: 691–700.

Berg RD. The indigenous gastrointestinal microflora. *Trends Microbiol.* 1996; (4): 430–435.

Bleich SN, Wolfson JA, Vine S, Wang YC. "Diet-beverage consumption and caloric intake among US adults, overall and by body weight." *Am J Public Health.* Mar 2014; 104 (3): 372–8. doi: 10.2105/AJPH.2013.301556. Epub Jan 16, 2014.

Bocarsly ME, Powell ES, Avena NM, Hoebel BG. "High-fructose corn syrup causes characteristics of obesity in rats: Increased body weight, body fat and triglyceride levels." *Pharmacol Biochem Behav.* Nov. 2010; 97 (1): 101–106.

Bray and Popkin BM. "Consumption of high-fructose corn syrup in beverages may play a role in the epidemic of obesity." 537–43.

Bray GA, Nielsen SJ, Popkin BM. "Consumption of high-fructose corn syrup in beverages may play a role in the epidemic of obesity." *Am J Clin Nutr.* Apr 2004; 79 (4): 537–43.

Bray GA, Ryan DH. "Drug treatment of the overweight patient." *Gastroenterology.* 2007; 132: 2239–52.

Bray GA. "How bad is fructose?" *Am Journal Clin Nutr.* 2007; 86 (4): 895–896.

Can S, Uysal C, Palaoğlu KE. "Short term effects of a low-carbohydrate diet in overweight and obese subjects with low HDL-C levels." BMC Endocr Disord. Nov. 9, 2010; 10: 18. doi: 10.1186/1472–6823–10–18.

Carnahan S, Balzer A, Panchal SK, Brown L. "Prebiotics in obesity." *Panminerva Med.* 2014; 56 (2): 165–75.

Center for Healthy Weight and Nutrition. *Motivational interviewing for weight-loss counseling in pediatric patients.* Nationwide children's pamphlet.

Centers for Disease Control and Prevention. Data and Statistics: Obesity Rates Among All Children in the United States [Internet]. Atlanta, GA: CDC; c2011 [cited May 27, 2012].

Chaput J, Drapeau V, Hetherington M, Lemieux S, Provencher V, Tremblay A. "Psychobiological effects observed in obese men experiencing body weight loss plateau." *Depress Anxiety.* 2007; 35: 518–21.

Cherala SS. "Gastric bypass surgeries in New Hampshire, 1996–1997." *Prev Chronic Dis.* 2012; 9:E72. Epub Mar 15, 2012.

Connolly HM, Crary JL, McGoon MD, Hensrud DD, Edwards BS, Edwards WD, Schaff HV. "Valvular Heart Disease Associated with Fenfluramine-Phentermine." *New Engl Journal Med.* Aug. 28, 1997; 337 (9): 581–8.

Connolly ML, Tuohy KM, Lovegrove JA. "Whole grain oat-based cereals have prebiotic potential and low glycemic index." *Br J Nutr.* 2012; 108 (12): 2198–206.

Cowley MA, Prortchuk N, Fan W, Dinulescu DM, Colmers WF, Cone RD. "Integration of NPY, AGRP, and Melanocortin Signals in the Hypothalamic Paraventricular Nucleus: Evidence of a Cellular Basis for the Adipostat." Neuron. 1999; 24: 155–63.

Dana Carpendar. *500 Paleo Recipes: Hundreds of Delicious Recipes for Weight Loss and Super Health.* Fair Winds Press.

DiNicolantonio JJ, O'Keefe JH, Lucan SC. "Added Fructose: A Principal Driver of Type 2 Diabetes Mellitus and Its Consequences." *Mayo Clin Proc.* Jan. 2015; pii: S0025–6196(15)00040–3. doi: 10.1016.

Djoussé L, Gaziano JM. "Alcohol consumption and heart failure: a systematic review." *Curr Atheroscler Rep.* Apr. 2008; 10 (2): 117–20.

Eastwood M, Kritchevsky D. "Dietary fiber: how did we get where we are?" *Annual Review Nutr.* 2005; 25: 1–8.

Elbel B, Kersh R, Brescoll VL, Dixon LB. "Calorie labeling and food choices: a first look at the effects on low-income people in New York City." *Health Aff (Millwood).* 2009 Nov–Dec; 28(6): w1110–21.

Elfhag K, Rossner S. "Who succeeds at maintaining weight loss? A conceptual review of factors associated with weight loss maintenance and weight regain." *Obes Rev.* 2005; 6:67–85.

ERS/USDA Briefing Room—"Sugar and Sweeteners: Background." United States Department of Agriculture. August 6, 2009.

Fairbrother K, Cartner B, Alley JR, Curry CD, Dickinson DL, Morris DM, Collier SR. "Effects of exercise timing on sleep architecture and nocturnal blood pressure in prehypertensives." *Vasc Health Risk Manag.* Dec 12, 2014; 10:691–8.

Feinman RD, Fine EJ. "Thermodynamics and metabolic advantage of weight loss diets." *Metab Syndr Relat Disord.* 2003; 1 (3): 209–219.

Fidler MC, Sanchez M, Raether B, Weissman NJ, Smith SR, Shanahan WR, Anderson CM; BLOSSOM Clinical Trial Group. "A one-year randomized trial of lorcaserin for weight loss in obese and overweight adults: the BLOSSOM trial." *Journal Clin Endocrinol Metab*. Oct. 2011; 96 (10): 3067–77.

Fildes A et al. "Probability of an Obese Person Attaining Normal Body Weight: Cohort Study Using Electronic Health Records." *Am Journal Public Health*. Jul. 16, 2015: e1–e6. [Epub ahead of print]

Flegal KD, Carroll MD, Kit BK, Ogden CL. "Prevalence of obesity and trends in the distribution of body mass index among US adults, 1999–2010." *JAMA*. 2012: 307(5): 491–497.

Flegal, Carroll, Kit, Ogden. "Prevalence of obesity and trends in the distribution of body mass index among US adults." 491–497.

Fortuna JL. "The obesity epidemic and food addiction: clinical similarities to drug dependence." *Journal Psychoactive Drugs*. 2012; 44 (1): 56–63.

Foster GD, Makris AP, Bailer BA. "Behavioral treatment of obesity." *Am Journal Clin Nutr*. 2005 Jul; 82 (1 Suppl): 230S–235S.

Foster GD, Wadden TA, Phelan S, Sarwer DB, Sanderson RS. "Obese patients' perceptions of treatment outcomes and the factors that influence them. *Arch Intern Med*. 2000; 161:2133–9.

Foster GD, Wadden TA, Vogt RA, Brewer G. "What is a reasonable weight loss? Patients' expectations and evaluations of obesity treatment outcomes." *Journal Consult Clin Psychol*. 1997; 65:79–85.

Foster-Powell K, Holt SG, Brand-Miller JC. (2002). "International Table of Glycemic Index and Glycemic Load Values: 2002." *Am Journal Clin Nutr*. 2002; 76 (1): 5–56.

Fowler SP, Williams K, Hazuda HP. "Diet Soft Drink Consumption Is Associated With Increased Waist Circumference in the San Antonio Longitudinal Study of Aging." (Paper presented at the American Diabetes Association, 71st Scientific Sessions, 2011). San Diego, Jun. 24–28, 2011 (Abstract Number: 62–OR).

Frank GK, Oberndorfer TA, Simmons AN, Paulus MP, Fudge JL, Kaye WH. "Sucrose Activates Human Taste Pathways Differently From Artificial Sweetener." *Neuroimage*. Feb. 2008; 39 (4): 1559–69. Epub Nov. 19, 2007.

Garvey WT, Ryan DH, Look M, Gadde KM, Allison DB, Peterson CA, Schwiers M, Day WW, Bowden CH. "Two-year sustained weight loss and metabolic benefits with controlled-release phentermine/topiramate in obese and overweight adults (SEQUEL): a randomized, placebo-controlled, phase 3 extension study." *Am J Clin Nutr.* 2012 Feb; 95 (2): 297–308. Epub Dec. 7, 2011.

Geier MS, Butler RN, Howarth GS. "Probiotics, prebiotics and synbiotics: a role in chemoprevention for colorectal cancer?" *Cancer Biol Ther.* Oct. 2006; 5 (10): 1265–1269.

Gilhooly C, Das S, Golden J, McCrory M, Dallal G, Saltzman E, Kramer F, Roberts S. "Food cravings and energy regulation: the characteristics of craved foods and their relationship with eating behaviors and weight change during 6 months of dietary energy restriction." *Int Journal Obes.* 2007; 31:1849–58.

Gloy VL et al. "Bariatric surgery versus non-surgical treatment for obesity: a systematic review and meta-analysis of randomized controlled trials." *BMJ.* 2013; 347: f5934. Published online October 22, 2013. doi: 10.1136/bmj.f5934

Goldman RL et al. "Executive control circuitry differentiates degree of success in weight loss following gastric-bypass surgery." *Obesity.* 2013 Nov; 21 (11): 2189–96.

Greenway FL, Fujioka K, Plodkowski RA, Mudaliar S, Guttadauria M, Erickson J, Kim DD, Dunayevich E, COR-I Study Group. "Effect of naltrexone plus bupropion on weight loss in overweight and obese adults (COR-I): a multicentre, randomised, double-blind, placebo-controlled, phase 3 trial." *Lancet.* Aug 21, 2010; 376 (9741): 595–605.

Guerrieri R, Nederkoorn C, Jansen A. "The interaction between impulsivity and a varied food environment: its influence on food intake and overweight." *Int Journal Obes (London).* Apr. 2008; 32 (4): 708–14.

Guerrieri R, Nederkoorn C, Schrooten M, Martijn C, Jansen A. "Inducing impulsivity leads high and low restrained eaters into overeating, whereas current dieters stick to their diet." *Appetite.* 2009 Aug; 53 (1): 93–100.

Gul A, Rahman MA, Hasnain SN. "Influence of fructose concentration on myocardial infarction in senile diabetic and non-diabetic patients." *Exp Clin Endocrinol Diabetes.* 2009; 17(10): 605–9.

Guthrie JF, Lin BH, Frazao E. "Role of food prepared away from home in the American diet, 1977–78 versus 1994–96: changes and consequences." *Journal Nutr Educ Behav.* 2002; 34: 140–150.

Hall KD. "Predicting metabolic adaptation, body weight change, and energy intake in humans." *Am J Physiol Endocrinol Metab.* 2010; 298: E449–66.

Hanover LM, White JS. "Manufacturing, Composition, and Application of Fructose." *Journal Clin Nutr.* 1993; 58: 724–732.

Havel PJ. "Dietary fructose: implications for dysregulation of energy homeostasis and lipid/carbohydrate metabolism." *Nutr Rev.* 2005; 63: 133–57.

Heacock PM, Hertzler SR, Wolf BW. "Fructose Prefeeding Reduces the Glycemic Response to a High-Glycemic Index, Starchy Food in Humans." *Journal Nutr.* 2002; 132 (9): 2601–2604.

Heisler LK, Chu HM, Tecott LH. "Epilepsy and obesity in serotonin 5–HT2C receptor mutant mice." *Ann N Y Acad Sci.* Dec. 15, 1998; 861: 74–8.

Hernandez TL, Kittelson JM, Law CK, Ketch LL, Stob NR, Lindstrom RC, Scherzinger A, Stamm ER, Eckel RH. "Fat redistribution following suction lipectomy: defense of body fat and patterns of restoration." *Obesity.* Jul. 2011; 19 (7):1388–95. Doi:10.1038/oby.2011.64. Epub Apr 7, 2011.

Hession M, Rolland C, Kulkarni U, Wise A, Broom J. "Systematic review of randomized controlled trials of low-carbohydrate vs. low-fat/low-calorie diets in the management of obesity and its comorbidities." *Obesity Rev.* 2009; 10:36–50.

Heymsfield SB, van Mierlo CAJ, van der Knaap HCM, Heo M, Frier HI. "Weight management using meal replacement strategy: meta and pooling analysis from six studies." *Int Journal Obes.* 2003; 27: 537–49.

Hoebel BG, Avena NM, Bocarsly ME, Rada P. "Natural addiction: a behavioral and circuit model based on sugar addiction in rats." *Addict Med.* Mar. 2009; 3 (1): 33–41.

Howard BV et al. "Low-fat dietary pattern and risk of cardiovascular disease: the Women's Health Initiative Randomized Controlled Dietary Modification Trial." *JAMA.* Feb. 9, 2006; 295(6): 655–66.

Howard BV, Manson JE, Stefanick ML, Beresford SA, Frank G, Jones B, Roadbough RJ, Snetselaar L, Thomson C, Tinker L, Vitolins M, Prentice R. "Low-fat dietary pattern and weight change over 7 years: the Women's Health Initiative Dietary Modification Trial." *JAMA.* Jan. 4, 2006; 295 (1): 39–49.

Hoyt G, Hickey MS, Cordain L. "Dissociation of the glycaemic and insulinaemic responses to whole and skimmed milk." *British Journal of Nutrition.* 2005 Feb; 93(2): 175–7

Iemolo A, Valenza M, Tozier L, Knapp CM, Kornetsky C, Steardo L, Sabino V, Cottone P. "Withdrawal from chronic, intermittent access to a highly palatable food induces depressive-like behavior in compulsive eating rats." *Behav Pharmacol.* Sept. 23, 2012; (5–6): 593–602.

Ikrumuddin SA et al. Effect of Reversible Intermittent Intra-abdominal Vagal Nerve Blockade on Morbid Obesity. The ReCharge Randomized Clinical Trial. *JAMA.* 2014; 312 (9):915–922.

Jansen A, Nederkoorn C, van Bakk L, Keirse C, Guerrieri R, Havermans R. "High-restrained eaters only overeat when they are also impulsive." *Behav Res Ther.* 2009 Feb; 47 (2): 105–10.

Jeffery RW, Wing RR, Thorson C, Burton LR. "Strengthening behavioral interventions for weight loss: a randomized trial of food provision and monetary incentives." *Journal Consult Clin Psychol.* 1993; 6:1038–45.

Jenkins DJ, Wong JM, Kendall CW, Esfahani A, Ng VW, Leong TC, Faulkner DA, Vidgen E, Paul G, Mukherjea R, Krul ES, Singer W. "Effect of a 6-month vegan low-carbohydrate ('Eco-Atkins') diet on cardiovascular risk factors and body weight in hyperlipidaemic adults: a randomised controlled trial." *BMJ Open.* Feb 5, 2014; 4 (2): e003505. doi: 10.1136/bmjopen-2013-003505.

Jequier E. Leptin."Signaling, adiposity, and energy balance." *Ann N Y Acad Sci.* 2002; 967: 379–88.

Kardas P. "Patient Compliance With Antibiotic Treatment For Respiratory Tract Infections." *Journal Antimicrob Agents.* 2002; 49: 897–903.

Kidwell B, Hasford J, Hardesty DM. "Emotional ability training and mindful eating." *Journal Mark Res.* 2014; 140723133331005 DOI: 10.1509/jmr.13.0188

King JC, Blumberg J, Ingwersen L, Jenab M, Tucker KL. "Tree nuts and peanuts as components of a healthy diet." *J Nutr.* 2008 Sep; 138 (9): 1736S–1740S.

Klein AV, Kiat H. "The mechanisms underlying fructose-induced hypertension: a review." *J Hypertens.* Feb. 2015. PMD 25715094.

Kremen AJ, Linner JH, Nelson CH. "An experimental evaluation of the nutritional importance of proximal and distal small intestine." *Ann Surg.* Sept. 1954; 140 (3): 439–48.

Latner JD, Stunkard AJ, Wilson GT, Jackson ML, Zelitch DS, Labouvie E. "Effective long term treatment of obesity: a continuing care model." *Int Journal Obes Relat Metab Disord.* Jul. 2000; 24 (7): 893–8.

Latner, J. D., Stukard, AJ. "Getting worse: the stigmatization of obese children." Obes Res. 2002 (11): 452–456.

Leathwood P, Pollet P. "Effects of slow release carbohydrates in the form of bean flakes on the evolution of hunger and satiety in man." *Appetite.* Feb. 1988; 10(1):1–11.

Leblanc ES, O'Connor E, Whitlock EP, Patnode CD, Kapka T. "Effectiveness of primary care-relevant treatments for obesity in adults: a systematic evidence review for the U.S. Preventive Services Task Force." *Ann Intern Med.* Oct. 4, 2011; 155 (7): 434–47.

Leibel RL, Rosenbaum M, Hirsch J. "Changes in energy expenditure resulting from altered body weight." *New Engl Journal Med.* 1995; 332 (10): 621–628.

Lericollais R, Gauthier A, Bessot N, Sesboue B, Davenne D. "Time-of-day effects on fatigue during a sustained anaerobic test in well-trained cyclists." *Chronobiol Int.* Dec 2009; 26(8):1622–35.

Lomax AR, Calder PC. "Prebiotics, immune function, infection and inflammation: a review of the evidence." *Br J Nutr.* Mar. 2009; 101 (5): 633–658.

Lucas KH, Kaplan-Machlis B. Orlistat—a novel weight loss therapy. *Ann Pharmacother.* 2001; 35: 314–28.

Luchsinger JA. "Diabetes, related conditions, and dementia." *Journal Neuro Sci.* Dec. 15, 2010; 299 (1–2).

Ludwig DS. "The glycemic index: physiological mechanisms relating to obesity, diabetes, and cardiovascular disease." *JAMA.* 2002; 287 (18): 2414–2423.

Lustig RH. "Fructose: Metabolic, Hedonic, and Societal Parallels with Ethanol." *Journal Am Diet Assoc.* Sept. 2010; 110 (9): 1307–21.

Maclean PS, Bergouignan A, Cornier Ma, Jackman MR. "Biology's response to dieting: the impetus for weight regain." *Am J Physiol Regul Integr Comp Physiol.* 2011; 301: R581–R600.

Madura JA, DiBaise JK. "Quick fix or long-term cure? Pros and cons of bariatric surgery." *F1000 Med Rep.* 2012; 4:19.

Malik VS, Schulze MB, Hu FB. "Intake of sugar-sweetened beverages and weight gain: A systematic review." *Am Journal Clin Nutr.* 2006; 84 (2): 274–88.

Marliss EB et al. "Glucagon levels and metabolic effects in fasting man." *J Clin Invest.* 1970; 49(12): 2256–2270. doi: 10.1172/JCI106445.

Martin CK, Rosenbaum D, Han H, Geiselman PJ, Wyatt HR, Hill JO, Brill C, Bailer B, Miller BV, Stein R, Klein S, Foster GD. "Change in Food Cravings, Food Preferences, and Appetite During a Low-Carbohydrate and Low-Fat Diet." *Obesity.* 2011; 19(10): 1963–70.

Metzgar CJ, Preston AG, Miller DL, Nickols-Richardson SM. "Facilitators and barriers to weight loss and weight loss maintenance: a qualitative exploration." *Journal Hum Nutr Diet.* 2014 Sept 18. doi: 10.1111/jhn.12273. [Epub ahead of print]

Michaelson R, Murphy DK, Gross TM, Whitcup SM; LAP-BAND Lower BMI Study Group. LAP-BANK for lower BMI: 2-year results from the multicenter pivotal study. *Obesity.* Jun. 2013; 21(6): 1148–58.

Miller WR, Rollnick S. *Motivational Interviewing: Preparing People for Change.* 2nd ed. New York, NY: Guilford Press; 2002.

Mozaffarian D, Hao T, Rimm EB, Willett WC, Hu FB. "Changes in Diet and Lifestyle and Long-Term Weight Gain in Women and Men." *New Engl Journal Med.* 2011; 364: 2392–404.

Mozaffarian D, Hao T, Rimm EB, Willett WC, Hu FB. Changes in Diet and Lifestyle and Long-Term Weight Gain in Women and Men. *New Engl Journal Med.* 2011; 364: 2392–404.

Muller MJ, Bosy-Westphal A, Heymsfield SB. "Is there evidence for a set point that regulates human body weight?" *F1000 Med Rep.* 2010; 2:59. Published online August 9, 2010. doi: 10.3410/M2-59

Murphy PW, Davis TC. "When low literacy blocks compliance." *RN.* 1997 Oct: 58–63.

Nabors LO. *American Sweeteners.* 2001. 374–375.

National Heart, Lung and Blood Institute. Bethesda, MD. 2000. NIH Publication No. 00–4084.

Nature. 2012 May 30; 485 (7400): 635–41. doi: 10.1038/nature11119.

Nederkoorn C, Braet C, Van Eijs Y, Tanghe A, Jansen A. "Why obese children cannot resist food: the role of impulsivity." *Eat Behav.* Nov. 2006; 7 (4): 315–22.

Neovius M, Johansson K, Rossner S. "Head-to-head studies evaluating efficacy of pharmaco-therapy for obesity: a systematic review and meta-analysis." *Obes Rev.* 2008; 9: 420–7.

Nguyen CT, Jensen B. "Implementation of a Diet Program for Inpatients with Schizophrenia." *Psychiatric Times.* Jan. 1, 2007. Vol. 24, No. 1.

Nguyen CT, Yu B.P., Maguire G.A. "Preemptive tactics to reduce weight gain." *Current Psychiatry* 2 (3), March 2003: 58–62.

Nichols-English G, Poirier S. "Optimizing adherence to pharmaceutical care plans." *Journal Am Pharm Assoc.* 2000; 40: 475–85.

O'Dea K, Nestel PJ, Antionoff L. "Physical factors influencing post-prandial glucose and insulin responses to starch." *Am Journal Clin Nutr.* 1980; 33: 760–5.

O'Neil PM. "Assessing dietary intake in the management of obesity." *Obes Res.* 2001; 9(suppl): 361S–6S.

O'Neil PM, Smith SR, Weissman NJ, Fidler MC, Sanchez M, Zhang J, Raether B, Anderson CM, Shanahan WR. "Randomized placebo-controlled clinical trial of lorcaserin for weight loss in type 2 diabetes mellitus: the BLOOM-DM study." Obesity (Silver Spring). Jul. 2012; 20(7): 1426–36. doi: 10.1038/oby.2012.66. Epub Mar 16, 2012.

Ohara T, Doi Y, Ninomiya T, Hirakawa Y, Hata J, Iwaki T, Kanba S, Kiyohara Y. "Glucose tolerance status and risk of dementia in the community: The Hisayama Study." *Neurology.* Sept. 20, 2011; 77(12): 1126–34.

Ott A, Stolk RP, van Harskamp F, Pols HA, Hofman A, Breteler MM. "Diabetes mellitus and the risk of dementia: The Rotterdam Study." *Neurology.* Dec. 10, 1999; 53 (9): 1937–42.

Parham ES. "Enhancing social support in weight loss management groups." *Journal Am Diet Assoc.* Oct. 1993; 93 (10): 1152–6.

Pereira MA, Kartashov AI, Ebbeling CB, et al. "Fast-food habits, weight gain, and insulin resistance (the CARDIA study): 15-year prospective analysis." *Lancet.* 2005; 365: 36–42.

Pollan M. "The (Agri)Cultural Contradictions Of Obesity," *New York Times*, October 12, 2003.

Putterman E, Linden W. "Appearance versus health: Does the reason for dieting affect dieting behavior?" *Journal Behav Med.* Apr 2004; 27 (2):185–204.

Raigond P, Ezekiel R, Raigond B. Resistant starch in food: a review. *Journal Sci Food Agric.* Oct. 2014; doi: 10.1002.

Rebello CJ et al. "Acute effect of oatmeal on subjective measures of appetite and satiety compared to a ready-to-eat breakfast cereal: a randomized crossover trial." *Journal Am Coll Nutr.* 2013; 32 (4): 272–9.

Roberts RO, Roberts LA, Geda YE, Cha RH, Pankratz VS, O'Connor HM, Knopman DS, Petersen RC. "Relative intake of macronutrients impacts risk of mild cognitive impairment or dementia." *Journal Alzheimers Dis.* 2012; 32 (2): 329–39. doi: 10.3233/JAD–2012–120862.

Roncal-Jimenez CA, Lanaspa MA, Rivard CJ, Nakagawa T, Sanchez-Lozada LG, Jalal D, Andres-Hernando A, Tanabe K, Madero M, Li N, Cicerchi C, Mc Fann K, Sautin YY, Johnson RJ. "Sucrose induces fatty liver and pancreatic inflammation in male breeder rats independent of excess energy intake." *Metabolism.* 2001; 60 (9): 1259–70.

Rorabaugh JM, Stratford JM, Zahniser NR. "A relationship between reduced nucleus accumbens shell and enhanced lateral hypothalamic orexin neuronal activation in long-term fructose bingeing behavior." *PLoS One.* Apr 15, 2014; 9 (4): e95019.

Rosenbaum M, Kissileff HR, Mayer LE, Hirsh J, Leibel RL. "Energy intake in weight-reduced humans." *Brain Res.* 2010; 1350:95–102.

Rosenbaum M, Leibe RL. "Adaptive thermogenesis in humans." *Int Journal Obes* (London). 2010 Oct; 34 (01): S47–S55.

Rothman RB, Baumann MH, Savage JE, Rauser L, McBride A, Hufeisen SJ, Roth BL. "Evidence for Possible Involvement of 5HT(2B) Receptors in the Cardiac Valuolpathy Associated with Fenfluramine and Other Serotonergic Medications." *Circulation.* Dec. 5, 2000; 102 (23): 2836–41.

Sackett DL, Haynes RB. Compliance with Therapeutic Regimens. John Hopkins University Press, London, UK (1976).

Sacks FM, Bray Ga, Carey VJ, et al. "Comparison of weight-loss diets with different compositions of fat, protein, and carbohydrates." *New Engl Journal Med.* 2009; 360: 859–73.

Scholz-Ahrens KE, Schrezenmeir J. "Insulin and oligofructose and mineral metabolism: the evidence from animal trials." *Journal Nutr.* 2007; 137(11 Supplements): 2513S–2523S.

Schwartz MB, Vartanian LR, Nosek BA, Brownell KD. "The Influence of One's Own Body Weight on Implicit and Explicit Anti-fat Bias." *Obesity.* Mar 14, 2006 (3): 440–47.

Scopinaro N, Adami GF, Marinari GM, Gianetta E, Traverso E, Friedman D, Camerini G, Baschieri G, Simonelli A. "Biliopancreatic diversion." *W J Surg.* Sept. 1998; 22 (9): 936–46.

Shukla AP, Iliescu RG, Thomas CE, Aronne LJ. "Food order has a significant impact on postprandial glucose and insulin levels." *Diabetes Care.* Jul 2015; 38(7):e98-9. doi: 10.2337/dc15-0429.

Smith SR, Weissman NJ, Anderson CM, Sanchez M, Chuang E, Stubbe S, Bays H, Shanahan WR; Behavioral Modification and Lorcaserin for Overweight and Obesity Management (BLOOM) Study Group. Multicenter, Placebo-Controlled Trial of Lorcaserin for Weight Management. *New Engl Journal Med.* Jul. 15, 2010; 363 (3): 245–56.

Soo-Jeong Kim, Dai-Jin Kim. "Alcoholism and Diabetes Mellitus." *Diabetes Metab J.* 2012; 36(2):108–115.

Stevens J, Levitsky DA, VanSoest PJ, Robertson JB, Kalkwarf HJ, Roe DA. "Effect of psyllium gum and wheat bran on spontaneous energy intake." *Am Journal Clin Nutr.* Nov. 1987; 46 (5):812–7.

Stuart RB. "Behavioral control of overeating." *Behav Ther.* 1967; 5: 357–65.

Sumithran P, Prendergast LA, Delbridge E, et al. "Long-term persistence of hormonal adaptations to weight loss." *New Engl Journal Med.* 2011; 365 (17): 1597–1604.

Teff KL, Elliott SS, Tschöp M, Kieffer TJ, Rader D, Heiman M, Townsend RR, Keim NL, D'Alessio D, Havel PJ. "Dietary fructose reduces circulating insulin and leptin, attenuates postprandial suppression of ghrelin, and increases triglycerides in women." *J Clin Endocrinol Metab.* Jun. 2004; 89 (6): 2963–72.

Thomas DM, Martin CK, Heymsfield SB, Redman LM, Schoeller DA, Levine JA. "A simple model predicting individual weight change in humans." *Journal Biol Dyn.* 2011; 5: 579–99.

Thomas DM, Martin CK, Redman LM, Heymsfield SB, Lettieri S, Levine JA, Bouchard C, Schoeller DA. "Effects of dietary adherence on the body weight plateau: a mathematical model incorporating intermittent compliance with energy intake prescription." *Am Journal Clin Nutrition.* 2014 Sep; 100 (3): 787–95.

Thorne MJ, Thompson LU, Jenkins DJ. "Factors affecting starch digestibility and the glycemic response with special reference to legumes." *Am Journal Clinical Nutr.* 1983; 38 (3):481–8.

Torgerson JS et al. "XENical in the prevention of diabetes in obese subjects (XENDOS) study: a randomized study of orlistat as an adjunct to lifestyle changes for the prevention of type 2 diabetes in obese patients." *Diabetes Care.* 2004; 27: 155–61.

Tsai AG, Wadden TA. "Systematic review: an evaluation of major commercial weight loss programs in the United States." *Ann Intern Med.* Jan. 4, 2005; 142 (1): 56–66.

Van Proeyen K, Szlufcik K, Nielens H, Pelgrim K, Deldicque L, Hesselink M, Van Veldhoven PP, Hespel P. "Training in the fasted state improves glucose tolerance during fat-rich diet." *Journal Physiol.* 2010 Nov 1; 588 (Pt 21): 4289–302.

Vartanian LR, Schwartz MB, Brownell KD. "Effects of soft drink consumption on nutrition and health: A systematic review and meta-analysis." *Am Journal Public Health.* 2007; 97 (4):667–75.

Wadden TA, Berkowitz RI, Sarwer DB, Prus-Wisniewski R, Steinberg C. "Benefits of lifestyle modification in the pharmacologic treatment of obesity: a randomized trial." *Arch Intern Med.* 2001; 161: 218–27.

Wadden TA, Foster GD. "Behavioral treatment of obesity." *Med Clin North Am. 2000; 84:* 441–61.

Wadden TA, Frey DL. "A multicenter evaluation of a proprietary weight loss program for the treatment of marked obesity: a five-year follow-up." *Int Journal of Eating Disord.* Sept. 22, 1997 (2): 203–12.

Wang YC, Bleich SN, Gortmaker SL. "Increasing caloric contribution from sugar-sweetened beverages and 100% fruit juices among US children and adolescents, 1988–2004." *Pediatrics.* 2008; 121 (6): e1604–e1614.

Webber KH, Tate DF, Ward DS, Bowling JM. "Motivation and its relationship to adherence to self-monitoring and weight loss in a 16-week Internet behavioral weight loss intervention." *Journal Nutr Educ Behav.* May–June, 2010; 42 (3): 161–7.

Weingarten HP, Elston D. "The phenomenology of food cravings."*Appetite.* 1990; 15: 231–246.

Werle CO, Wansink B, Payne CR. "Is it fun or exercise? The framing of physical activity biases subsequent snacking." *Mark Lett.* May 15, 2014. DOI 10.1007/s11002–014–9301–6.

Wesseler J, Scatasta S, Nillesen E. "The Maximum Incremental Social Tolerable Irreversible Costs (MISTICs) and other Benefits and Costs of Introducing Transgenic Maize in the EU-15." *Pedobiologia.* 2007; 51 (3): 261–269.

Wing RR, Jeffery RW, Burton LR, Thorson C, Nissinoff KS, Baxter JE. "Food provision vs structured meal plans in the behavioral treatment of obesity." *Int Journal Obes Relat Metab Disord.* 1996; 20: 56–62.

Wing RR, Jeffery RW. "Benefits of recruiting participants with friends and increasing social support for weight loss and maintenance." *Journal Consult Clin Psychol.* Feb. 1999; 67 (1):132–138.

Wing RR, Lang W, Wadden TA, Safford M, Knowler WC, Bertoni AG, Hill JO, Brancati FL, Peters A, Wagenknecht L; Look AHEAD Research Group. "Benefits of modest weight loss in improving cardiovascular risk factors in overweight and obese individuals with type 2 diabetes." *Diabetes Care.* Jul. 2011; 34 (7):148–6.

Wolever T, Bolognesi C. "Time of day influences relative glycemic effect of foods." *Nutrition Research.* Mar. 1996; 16 (3): 381–384.

Wolfe WA. "A review: maximizing social support—a neglected strategy for improving weight management with African-American women." *Ethn Dis.* 2004 Spring; 14 (2): 212–8.

World Health Organization. "Adherence to long-term therapies: evidence for action." (2003). www.who.int/chp/knowledge/publications/adherence_full_report.pdf

Yoon YS, Oh SW, Baik HW, Park HS, Kim WY. "Alcohol consumption and the metabolic syndrome in Korean adults: the 1998 Korean National Health and Nutrition Examination Survey." *Am J Clin Nutr.* Jul. 2004; 80 (1): 217–24.

Zatu MC, Van Rooyen JM, Kruger A, Schutte AE. "Alcohol intake, hypertension development and mortality in black South Africans." *Eur Journal Prev Cardiol.* Dec 2014; pii: 2047487314563447.

WEBSITES

www.ama-assn.org/ama/pub/news/news/2013/2013-06-18-new-ama-policies-annual-meeting.page

www.ars.usda.gov/is/ar/archive/jun00/sugar0600.pdf

www.aspartame.org

www.bmc.org/nutritionweight/services/weightmanagement.htm

http://www.cmsa.org/portals/0/pdf/CMAG2.pdf

www.ers.usda.gov/briefing/potatoes/

www.ers.usda.gov/Data/FoodConsumption/

www.ers.usda.gov/media/134674/tb1927.pdf

www.fda.gov/downloads/advisorycommittees/committeesmeetingmaterials/drugs/endocrinologicandmetabolicdrugsadvisorycommittee/ucm235671.pdf

www.foodnavigator-usa.com/Product-Categories

https://my.americanheart.org/idc/groups/ahamah-public/@wcm/@sop/@
smd/documents/downloadable/ucm_425988.pdf

www.neotame.com

www.nutritionexpress.com/article+index/vitamins+supplements+a-z
/showarticle.aspx?id=120

www.odi.org/news/703-overweight-obese-adults-reaching-almost-billion
-developing-countries-as-numbers-continue-grow-richer-nations

www.plasticsurgery.org/cosmetic-procedure

www.quorn.com

www.saccharin.org

www.stevia.com

www.sucralose.org

www.washingtonpost.com/blogs/wonkblog/wp/2015/02/10/feds-poised
-to-withdraw-longstanding-warnings-about-dietary-cholesterol/

www.webmd.com/diet/20090615/skip-breakfast-get-fat

www.who.int/mediacentre/factsheets/fs394/en/

www.wildwoodfoods.com/

Index

AACE. *See* American Association of Clinical Endocrinologists
ACC. *See* American College of Cardiology
acesulfame potassium, 60
Active Phase
  eating five times per day, 15–16, 89, 179
  fiber for, 54
  GI and GL during, 53
  insulin in, 132, 170
  overview, 67–71, 128–130, 128 (fig.), 129 (fig.)
  processed foods and, 45
  starving avoided, 89
  staying on track, 19
  temptations during, 18
  transitioning from, 114
  weight-loss during, 170
Active Phase, exercise
  aerobics, Zumba, yoga, 101–102
  carbohydrates and, 100
  for minimizing weight gain, 147
  motivation for, 99
  overview, 99–100
  self-monitoring tools, 104
  success stories, 102, 103 (photo), 104
  walking, 101

Active Phase, food groups
  avoiding grains, 80–81
  establishing food groups, 76–88
  fruits, 78–80
  overview, 73–76
  proteins, 84–88
  red, yellow, green lights, 87–88, 87 (fig.)
  summary, 88
  sweets, 76–78
  vegetables, 81–84
Active Phase, meal plans
  avoid starving self, 89
  breakfast, 90–92
  eating five times per day, 89
  example 1, 95–96
  example 2, 96
  example 3, 96–97
  lunches and dinners, 93–95
  morning and afternoon snacks, 92–93
  overview, 89–90
  portion sizes, 90
Active Phase, milestones
  cheating and, 117–118
  eating five times per day, 115
  grouping foods in five categories, 115–117
  red, yellow, green lights, 116–117

Active Phase, milestones *(continued)*
  week 2, 116
  week 3, 116–117
  week 4, 117
  weeks 5–8, 117
  weeks 9–12, 117–118
  weeks 13–17, 118
ADA. *See* American Diabetic
  Association
adaptive thermogenesis, 126
adenosine triphosphate (ATP),
  25–26, 86
adherence
  Adherence Intention box,
    158–159, 159 (table)
  defined, 157
  level for staying on track, 158–159
  long-term, 158
Adipex-P®, 212
adipose tissue, 31, 31 (fig.), 210
Adipost®, 212
aerobics, 101–102
AHA. *See* American Heart
  Association
alcohol
  fructose and, 59
  grains and, 190
  hypertension and, 59
  insulin and, 189–190
  Thinsulin Program and, 189–190
Alli®, 211
all-or-nothing thinking, 12, 87
  absolute terms in, 108
  caught in, 19–20
  CBT and, 68
  challenging, 109
  falling into, 148
  negative thinking, 112
  as obstacle to change, 111
alpha bonds, 44–45

Alzheimer's disease, 29–30
AMA. *See* American Medical
  Association
American Association of Clinical
  Endocrinologists (AACE), 4,
  208
American College of Cardiology
  (ACC), 208
American Diabetic Association
  (ADA), 216
American Dream, xiv, 187
American Heart Association (AHA),
  82, 208
American Journal of Clinical Nutrition,
  45, 54, 127
American Journal of Public Health, 4
American Medical Association
  (AMA), 4
American Society of Bariatric
  Physicians (ASBP), 208
American Society of Metabolic and
  Bariatric Surgery, 227
amphetamines, 212
Angelou, Maya, 10
Anorex-SR®, 212
Appecon®, 212
appetite, 16–17
  controlling, 209–210
  hunger and, 210
  medications for suppression,
    212–214
  reducing, 141
  sleep and, 201
  See also satiety
apples, 79, 90, 115, 138, 204
Arena Pharmaceuticals, 215
Aronne, Louis, 4, 141
artificial sweeteners, 77, 185
  acesulfame potassium, 60
  aspartame, 60

benefits, 62
carbohydrates and, 60–64
neotame, 61
saccharin, 61
stevia, 61
sucralose, 60–61
sugar cravings and, 62–64
See also specific sweeteners
arugula, 191, 193
ASBP. *See* American Society of
    Bariatric Physicians
asparagus, 82, 191
aspartame, 60
aspartic acid, 60
Atkins, Robert C., 191
Atkins diet, xvii, 9, 125
    phases of, 191
    Thinsulin Program compared to,
        190–191
ATP. *See* adenosine triphosphate
Avena, Nicole M., 57
avocados, 79, 95, 191

bananas, 45, 78, 79, 91, 111, 138
bariatric surgery, 224–227
barley, 80, 136, 204
basal metabolic rate, 130
BPD-DS. *See* duodenal switch
beans, 85–87, 195, 196
Beck, Aaron T., 108
beef, 84–85, 94, 115, 194–195, 202
beer bellies, 81, 189
beets, 81, 83, 115, 137, 159, 204
behavioral modification, 168
behavioral therapy, 168–169
    goal setting and, 169–172
    self-monitoring and, 172–173, 175
    See also Cognitive Behavioral
        Therapy
Belviq®, 208, 215–216

berries, 79, 90, 115, 138, 204
beta bonds, 44
bicycling, 149
biliopancreatic diversion (BPD),
        226–227
bingeing, 121, 178, 184
biopsychosocial approach, 104, 106,
        169, 183
bipolar disorder, xiv, xv
blackberries, 79, 115
blood glucose
    insulin regulation, 26–28,
        27 (fig.), 32
    levels for cell life, 25–26
    normal levels, 34
    stress and, 28
blueberries, 79, 115
BMI. *See* Body Mass Index
body contouring, 230–231
Body Mass Index (BMI), 3, 6, 35,
        173, 184
    decreasing, 9, 213
    obese, 198
bok choy, 82
Bontril PDM®, 212
Bontril SR®, 212
BPD. *See* biliopancreatic diversion
brachioplasty, 230–231
brain
    basal ganglia, 167
    dopamine receptors, 167, 178
    glucose and, 57–58
    glycogen and, 31–32, 31 (fig.)
    hypothalamus, 210, 216, 218
    insulin and, 28–30
    intense desire and, 180
    nucleus accumbens, 58
    opioid receptors, 178
    oxygen and, 55
    prefrontal cortex, 179, 180

brain *(continued)*
　reward system, 62–63, 167, 178
　signaling, 219–220
　tricking, 77
　unconscious neurobehavioral
　　processes, 177, 179, 181
breakfast
　in Active Phase meal plans, 90–92
　hunger and, 91
　proteins for, 91–92
　reducing hunger, 91
　what to eat, 202–203
breast augmentation surgery, 229
British Journal of Medicine, 195
broccoli, 137, 191, 194
buffet dinners, 96, 124
bupropion, 218–219
Burger King®, 106

calories
　body using, 200
　control of, xvii
　defined, 37
　empty, 57–58, 77
　insulin and, 188
　Passive Phase exercise and,
　　147–148
　posted for fast foods, 106
　reducing, 125
　sugar in SAD, 37–38
　weight-loss emphasis, xvii–xviii
cancer, 185, 217
cantaloupes, 78
carbohydrates, 27 (fig.)
　Active Phase exercise and, 100
　artificial sweeteners and, 60–64
　control of, 131, 139
　as enjoyment food, 134
　fiber and, 53–55
　fructose and HFCS, 55–60

GI and, 46–53
insulin and, 25
overview and definitions,
　43–44
SAD and, 40–42
starch and glycogen, 44–46
traditional eating, 68
See also Passive Phase,
　carbohydrates and
carrots, 81, 83, 96–97, 115,
　137–138, 159
cauliflower, 70, 82, 194
CBT. *See* Cognitive Behavioral
　Therapy
CDC. *See* Centers for Disease
　Control and Prevention
celery, 82, 93, 96, 159, 194, 202
Cell journal, 211
cellulose, 44, 53, 191
　See also fiber
Centers for Disease Control and
　Prevention (CDC), 37, 224
changing thinking
　CBT for, 108–112, 114
　concepts for, 107
　from "I enjoy eating" to "I eat for
　　enjoyment," 151
　overview, 105–108
　for weight loss, xix–xx
　during weight-loss journey,
　　21–22
　See also all-or-nothing thinking
Chantix®, 208
cheating
　Active Phase milestones and,
　　117–118
　insulin and, 33–34, 170
　myths about weight-loss journey,
　　18–19
　preventing, 180

cherries, 79, 115
chicken, 36–37, 84, 88, 90, 115
  broiled, 173
  broth, 202
  for energy, 149
  grilling, 141–142, 194–195
classical conditioning, 168
club soda, 77, 192
Cognitive Behavioral Therapy
    (CBT), xx
  all-or-nothing thinking and, 68
  for changing habits, 73, 106
  for changing thinking, 108–113,
    114
  development of, 108
  identifying faulty thoughts,
    110–111
  principles, 73, 106
  psychology of, 169, 187
Collier, S. R., 149
comfort foods, 21, 28, 68, 180
compliance, 157–158
Contrave™, 208, 217–219
control, 186
  appetite, 209–210
  of calories, xvii
  of carbohydrates, 131, 139
  enjoyment and, 21–22
  of food cravings, 10, 77, 108
  lack of, 110
  of life, 176
  out-of-control, 121
  self-control, 110, 134, 177
  weight, 67, 74, 97, 163,
    172, 205
  See also inhibitory control
corn, 56, 81, 96–97, 115, 137, 204
cortisol, 130–131
cranberries, 115, 160, 190
cucumbers, 77, 82, 93

dairy products
  cheese, 68, 85, 90–91, 202
  yogurt, 85, 90, 202
dancing, 148
Davis, William, 80–81
depression, xiv, 3
  active, 228
  negative beliefs and, 108–109
  obesity and, 220
desserts, 68, 77–78, 123–124
destructive thought patterns, 109
dexfenfluramine, 214
diabetes, xv, 14, 25, 170
  gestational, 205
  Thinsulin Program and,
    203–204
  Types 1 and 2, 28, 57, 59,
    203–204, 215–217, 224
Diabetes Care, 141
diethylpropion, 213
diets
  diet sodas, 62–63
  fad, 74
  Jenny Craig, 125
  low-fat, 39–40
  Mediterranean, 125
  myths about weight-loss journey,
    15–16
  WIN-Nguyen, xvii–xviii
  See also Atkins diet; Paleo diet;
    standard American diet; Weight
    Watchers®
dinners
  in Active Phase meal plans,
    93–95
  buffet, 96, 124
  meats for, 93, 95
  sauces and condiments, 94
disaccharides, 44, 55
domino effect, 159

dopamine receptors, 167, 178
duck, 84
Duhigg, Charles, 167
dumping syndrome, 226
duodenal switch (BPD-DS), 227

eating for enjoyment, 20–22, 151
eating out, 140–141, 160
  buffet dinners, 96, 124
Eckel, Robert, 229
egg whites, 84–85, 88, 90, 115, 149, 196, 202
Eisai Inc., 215
electrolytes, 126
empathy, 162, 164
empty calories, 57–58, 77
enjoyment food
  carbohydrates as, 134
  changing thinking from "I enjoy eating" to "I eat for enjoyment," 151
  insulin increased with, 22, 138
  overeating, 152
  in Passive Phase, 123–124, 152
  in Passive Phase carbohydrates, 134–136, 139–145
  in Passive Phase exercise, 148
  selecting, 132
EnteroMedics, 219
epilepsy, 217
Equal®, 60
exercise
  aerobics, 101–102
  bicycling, 149
  dancing, 148
  kickboxing, 100, 148
  running, 149
  swimming, 149
  walking, 101, 116
  yoga, 101, 148
  Zumba, 101–102
  See also Active Phase, exercise; Passive Phase, exercise

Facebook, Thinsulin Program page, 160
fad diets, 74
fast foods, 36–37, 70
  calorie posting, 106
fasting, 197, 210
  blood sugar levels, 216
  fasting insulin, 32, 34
fat, 58
  burning, 153, 187
  fat cells, 31 (fig.)
  fatty acids, 33 (fig.)
  low-fat diets, 39–40
  metabolism, 122
  saturated fats, 39
  short-chain fatty acids, 54
  storing in body, 127
FDA. See Food and Drug Administration
Federal Trade Commission (FTC), 213
feedback, 175–176
fenfluramine, 214–215
fen-phen, 196, 214
fiber, 44
  for Active and Passive Phases of Thinsulin Program, 54
  carbohydrates and, 53–55
  GI and, 54–55
  GL and, 54
  insoluble, 54–55
  soluble, 53–54
fight-or-flight response, 28
fish, 84, 94, 115, 173, 194

Food and Drug Administration
(FDA), 61–62, 208, 213–217,
219
food cravings, xvi–xvii, 127
control of, 10, 77, 108
food rewards and, 178–179
hard-wired, 178
inhibitory control and, 178–179
medications for, 182
night eating and, 200
overview, 177–178
playing defense, 181
sugar, 70, 168, 185–186
sweets, 63, 139
time discounting and, 180–182
tracking, 173
unconscious neurobehavioral
processes, 177
food diaries, 172–173
food groups
breaking into five, 159
excluding, 14
of food pyramid, 40
See also Active Phase, food groups;
fruits; grains; proteins; sweets;
vegetables
food logs, 116, 160, 172–173
food pictures, 117, 160
food plans, 169
food pyramid, 73, 105
food groups of, 40
food rewards
food cravings and, 178–179
science of, 178
solution, 178–179
fructose, 38, 43–44
alcohol and, 59
GI and, 55
glycogen and, 58
HFCS and, 55–60

liver disease and, 59
fruits, 115, 191
in Active Phase food groups,
78–80
apples, oranges, grapes, berries as
mantra, 79
high-and low-GI, 78–79
low-GI fruit for morning snack,
92
in Passive Phase carbohydrates,
138
portions, 79
as snacks, 78–79
See also specific fruits
FTC. *See* Federal Trade
Commission
Fusarium venenatum, 195

galactose, 43–44
gastric bypass, 227–228
gastric sleeve, 225–226
genetics, 169
gestational diabetes, 205
ghrelin, 58, 210
GI. *See* Glycemic Index
GL. *See* Glycemic Load
glaucoma, 217
GLP-1. *See* glucagon-like peptide-1
glucagon, 26, 210–211
glucagon-like peptide-1 (GLP-1),
210–211
glucose
brain and, 57–58
energy source, 57
foods converting to, 46
insulin and, 46
metabolizing, 43
need for, 26
starch and, 44
See also blood glucose

Glycemic Index (GI), 30
for 100+ foods, 47–52 (table)
during Active and Passive
Phases, 53
carbohydrates and, 46–53
fiber and, 54–55
fructose and, 55
fruits in, 78–79
low in Passive Phase, 130–131
overview, 46–47
starch on, 45
Glycemic Load (GL)
for 100+ foods, 47–52 (table)
during Active and Passive
Phases, 53
calculating, 47
fiber and, 54
of grains, 80
glycogen, 26
brain and, 31–32, 31 (fig.)
fructose and, 58
starch and, 44–46
goals
setting, 169–172
shifts, 123
starving and, 68
weight loss, 68–70
Goldman, Rachel, 228–229
grains, 115
alcohol and, 190
avoiding in Active Phase food
groups, 80–81
barley, 80, 136, 204
GL of, 80
oats, 80, 136, 204
obesity and, 81
Passive Phase carbohydrates,
136–137
quinoa, 81, 136, 204
rice, 80, 136
wheat, 81–82, 136, 204

grapes, 79, 81, 90, 115, 138, 189
green tea, 213

habits
altering, xix
breaking bad, xx, 5, 167–176
CBT for changing, 73, 106
eating, 8, 9, 12, 108
feedback and reinforcement,
175–176
goal setting and, 169–172
habit loop for, 167–168
new for Passive Phase, 19, 131
overeating, 167
overview, 167–169
self-monitoring and, 172–173, 175
triggers, 168, 172
hazelnuts, 86
health literacy, 158
heart, 57
heart healthy, 99
heart rate, 119, 226
heart disease, 25, 45, 59, 94, 204, 226
hemoglobin A1C, 216
Herbalife shakes, 125
herbs, 193
HFCS. See high-fructose corn syrup
high cholesterol, xv, 59, 215–217, 226
high-fructose corn syrup (HFCS),
36–37
derivation from corn, 56
fructose and, 55–60
hunger and, 58
obesity and, 56–57
in tonic water, 192
Hoebel, Bartley G., 57, 178
homeostasis, 20, 123, 126, 127
hunger, 5
appetite and, 210
breakfast and, 91
fighting, 15

fulfilling, 110
increasing, 126
monitoring, 173, 175
satisfying, 201
snacks and, 84
targeting with pharmacotherapy, 209
hyperinsulinemia, 30, 215–216
hypertension, 25, 170, 217
alcohol and, 59
hyperthyroidism, 212, 217
hypoglycemia, 26, 203–204
hypothalamus, 210, 216, 218
hypothermia, 212

inhibitory control
food cravings and, 179–180
science of, 179
solution, 179–180
starving and, 179–180
stress and, 179
insoluble fiber, 54–55
insulin, 27 (fig.), 31 (fig.), 33 (fig.)
in Active Phase, 132, 170
alcohol and, 189–190
biology of, 106, 114, 187
blood glucose regulation, 26–28, 27 (fig.), 32
brain and, 28–30
calories and, 188
carbohydrates and, 25
cheating and, 33–34, 170
deficiencies and disease, 28–30
enjoyment food increasing, 22, 138
fasting, 32, 34
food in terms of, 111
glucose and, 46
hyperinsulinemia, 30, 215–216
as magic hormone, 6

nutrition knowledge compared to, 185
overview, 25–26
in Passive Phase, 131–133, 171
regulating blood glucose, 26–28, 27 (fig.), 32
resistance, 29–30
science of, 112, 122
spiking, 78, 88, 112, 132, 176, 181
thinking in terms of, 95
weight management and, 30–32, 31 (fig.), 33 (fig.)
weight-loss and, xiii, xviii, 183
Ionamin®, 212

Jenny Craig®, 125
Johns Hopkins University, 61
Journal of Alzheimer's Disease, 29–30
Journal of Marketing Research, 180
Journal of Nutrition, 86
Journal of the American Dietetic Association, 177
Journal of the American Medical Association, 130
junk food, 20, 38, 87, 110, 196
avoiding, 77, 177
prescription medications and, 208–209

kale, 54, 82, 159, 191, 193–194
Kardas, P., 107
Kentucky Fried Chicken®, 106
kickboxing, 100, 148
kidneys, 57

lactose, 44
lacto-vegetarians, 195
LAL. *See* laser-assisted liposuction
LAP-BAND® System, 225–226
laser-assisted liposuction (LAL), 229

lemons, 193–194
leptin, 58, 210
lettuce, 82, 93, 143, 160, 193
lipase, 212
liposuction, 229–230
liver, 31 (fig.), 190
long-term adherence, 158
lorcaserin, 215
Lorphen Medical Clinic, 5, 40, 67, 111, 122, 175
low-fat diets, 39–40
Luchsinger, Jose, 30
lunches
    in Active Phase meal plans, 93–95
    meats for, 93, 95
    sauces and condiments, 94
    vegetables and proteins for, 93–94

Maestro® Rechargeable System, 219–220
magnesium, 82, 86–87
Maimonides, 105
malabsorption, 226–228
maladaptive behaviors, 168
Marketing Letters, 101
Mayo Clinic, 214
McDonald's, 106
MCI. *See* mild cognitive impairment
meal plans. *See* Active Phase, meal plans
meal replacements, 169
meats, 8, 76, 84, 88, 115–116
    fatty, 39
    increasing, 85
    lean, 149, 152, 191
    for lunches and dinners, 93, 95
    preparing, 94
    red, 57, 83
    See also specific meats

medications
    antipsychotic, xvi–xvii
    for appetite suppression, 212–214
    brain signaling and, 219–220
    for breaking obesity cycle, 220–221
    for food cravings, 182
    increasing satiety, 214–220
    junk food and, 208–209
    nutrient absorption interference and, 211–212
    overview, 207–209
    regulation of food intake and, 209–211
Mediterranean diet, 125
Melfiat®, 213
mental illness, 205
mentorship, 166
Meridia®, 215
mesolimbic reward pathways, 218
metabolic syndrome, xv, 59, 224
metabolism, 18, 59, 122, 169, 212
methanol, 60
MI. *See* motivational interviewing
migraines, 185, 197, 217
mild cognitive impairment (MCI), 29–30
mind-body connection, xix, 9
mineral water, 192
Mintel, 60
monoamine oxidase inhibitors, 217
monosaccharides, 43, 46
MORs. *See* mu-opioid receptors
motivation, 8, 207
    for Active Phase exercise, 99
    to make changes, 157
    overeating and, 164
    social support and, 165
    success and, 22
    for weight loss, 14–15, 122, 158

motivational interviewing (MI)
  empathy and, 162, 164
  engage, 162–163
  evoke response, 162–164
  focus, 162–163
  plan, 162, 164
  for staying on track, 161–165
mu-opioid receptors (MORs), 211
Murphy's Law, 180
muscles, 31 (fig.), 57, 100
mushrooms, 82
Mycoprotein, 195
myths about weight-loss journey
  cheating doesn't matter, 18–19
  dieting, 15–16
  eating for enjoyment, 20–22
  no point in continuing, 19–20
  no time to eat, 16–17

naltrexone, 218
National Cancer Institute, 62
National Health and Nutrition
    Examination Surveys
    (NHANES), 39, 57
National Heart, Lung, and Blood
    Institute (NHLBI), 208
National Lipids Association (NLA),
    208
negative reinforcement, 169
neotame, 61
neurological loop, 167–168
New England Journal of Medicine, 82,
    214
NHANES. *See* National Health and
    Nutrition Examination Surveys
NHLBI. *See* National Heart, Lung,
    and Blood Institute
night eating, 200–201
night workers, 201–202
NLA. *See* National Lipids Association

noncompliance, 107
NuNaturals, 61
NutraSweet®, 60
NutriSystem, 125
nutrition
  claims, 88
  deficiencies, 227
  education, 106
  evaluation, 228
  experts, 25, 39, 55, 80
  healthy practices, xvii
  insulin knowledge compared to,
    185
nuts, 85, 191
  almonds, 86, 93
  hazelnuts, 86
  peanuts, 87
  pecans, 86
  pistachios, 93
  for snacks, 92–93, 179–180, 201
  walnuts, 86

oats, 80, 136, 204
obesity
  causes, 4
  depression and, 220
  in developing world, 36
  grains and, 81
  HFCS and, 56–57
  medications for breaking cycle,
    220–221
  perception of, 207
  rates and attitude toward, 3–4
  SAD and, 35–37
  science of, xv–xvii
  struggle against, 8
  Thinsulin Program for fighting
    epidemic, 187
  treatment of, xiii, 162
  See also overweight

Obesity journal, 225, 229
The Obesity Society (TOS), 9, 208
Obezine®, 213
oils, 86, 93, 194
operant conditioning, 168–169
opioid receptors, 178
oranges, 79, 90, 115, 138, 204
Orexigen Therapeutics, Inc., 217
Orlistat, 211–212
overeating, 19, 63, 67–68, 141
   avoiding, 91
   enjoyment food, 152
   habits, 167
   motivation and, 164
   preventing, 92
   skipping meals and, 200
   unconscious neurobehavioral
      processes and, 177
Overseas Development Institute, 36
overweight
   defined, 3
   in developing world, 36
   sugary drinks and, 57
oxygen, 55

Paleo diet, 9
   mimicking hunter gatherers,
      190–191
   Thinsulin Program compared to,
      190–191
pancreas, 27 (fig.), 211
   beta cells, 26, 28, 33
   break down of, 29
pancreatitis, 59
paradigm shift, 187–188
parsnips, 82
Passive Phase, xviii–xix
   eating five times per day, 16, 131,
      151
   eating for enjoyment, 22

   enjoyment food in, 123–124,
      152
   fiber for, 54
   GI and GL during, 53
   goal shifts, 123
   insulin in, 131–133, 171
   mentorship and, 166
   new habits for, 19, 131
   overview, 121–124, 128–130,
      128 (fig.), 129 (fig.)
   processed foods and, 45
   start of, 126
   transitioning to, 114
   troubleshooting, 122
   weighing in, 19, 142, 144–145,
      153, 173
Passive Phase, carbohydrates and
   in clinical practice, 142–145
   enjoyment food, 134–136,
      139–145
   fruits and, 138
   grains and, 136–137
   overview, 133
   reintroducing, 134
   sweets, 138–140
   vegetables and, 137–138
   week 17, 134–140
   weeks 17-29, 134 (table)
   when to eat carbohydrates,
      140–141
Passive Phase, exercise, 123
   calories and, 147–148
   enjoyment food in, 148
   overview, 147–148
   types, length, frequency of exercise,
      148
   when to exercise, 148–149
Passive Phase, milestones
   week 29, 153
   weeks 17-20, 151–152

weeks 21-24, 152
weeks 25-28, 153
Passive Phase, weight-loss plateau and
   low GI as best, 130–131
   overview, 125–128
   raising insulin, 131–132
Paulus, Martin P., 63
peaches, 138
pears, 138
pedometers, 104
peppers, 82
peptides, 211
*Pharmacology, Biochemistry and
   Behavior,* 57
pharmacotherapy, 169, 205, 208–209,
   211, 215
   See also medications
Phendiet®, 213
phendimetrazine, 212–213
Phenmetrazine, 212–213
phentermine, 208, 212–213, 214
   See also fen-phen
phenylalanine, 60
phosphorus, 86
photosynthesis, 26, 43
pineapple, 45, 78, 111, 138
plastic surgery, 229, 230
Plegine®, 213
polysaccharides, 44, 191
pork, 84, 94, 202
positive reinforcement, 168–169
potatoes, 81–83, 96–97, 115, 137, 204
*The Power of Habit: Why We Do What
   We Do In Life and Business*
   (Duhigg), 167
prebiotics, 54
prefrontal cortex, 179, 180
pregnancy, 204–205, 217
Prelu-2®, 213
Preludin®, 212

preparing vegetables, 193–194
Princeton University, 57, 178
processed foods, 45, 55–56, 60, 79
proteins, 115
   in Active Phase food groups,
      84–86
   beans, 85–87, 195, 196
   beef, 84–85, 94, 115, 194–195, 202
   for breakfast, 91–92
   cheese, 68, 85, 90–91, 202
   common sense and, 84
   for dinners, 93–94
   duck, 84
   egg whites, 84–85, 88, 90, 115,
      149, 196, 202
   fish, 84, 94, 115, 173, 194
   for lunches, 93–94
   Mycoprotein, 195
   pork, 84, 94, 202
   seafood, 84–85, 88, 94, 115, 194
   tofu, 84–87, 94
   turkey, 84, 88, 94, 115, 195
   yogurt, 85, 90, 202
   See also chicken; meats; nuts
psychiatry
   weight gain with antipsychotic
      drugs, xv–xvi, 74
   weight loss and, xv
psychology, 14, 169, 187
punishment-reward-guilt cycle, 68

Qsymia®, 208, 217
quinoa, 81, 136, 204
Quorn™, 195

radishes, 82
raisins, 79
raspberries, 79, 115
Redux®, 214
REE. *See* resting energy expenditure

reinforcement, 175–176
resting energy expenditure (REE), 130
restriction, 227–228
ReVia®, 218
rewards, 169
rice, 80, 136
Rothman, R. B., 214
Roux-en-Y gastric bypass, 227–228
running, 149
Ryun, Jim, 167

sabotage, 166
    self-sabotage, 67, 179
saccharin, 61
SAD. *See* standard American diet
SAL. *See* suction-assisted liposuction
salads, 81, 93, 96, 160
satiety
    combination medications and, 217–219
    medications for increasing, 214–220
saturated fats, 39
sauces and condiments, 78, 94
Saxenda®, 208, 211, 216–217
schizophrenia, xv–xvi, 162
SCOUT. *See* Sibutramine Cardiovascular Outcomes
seafood, 84–85, 88, 94, 115, 194
Sears, Barry, 125
self-control, 110, 134, 177
self-esteem, 121
self-monitoring, 104, 172–173, 175
self-reflection, 165
seltzer water, 77, 192
serotonin, 205
serotonin 5-HT system, 214–216
short-chain fatty acids, 54
sibutramine, 215

Sibutramine Cardiovascular Outcomes (SCOUT), 215
Skinner, B. F., 168–169
skipping meals, 17, 19, 91, 179, 200, 201
sleep, 201
Slim-Fast shakes, 125
Slimlipo™, 229
Smartlipo™, 229
snacks
    in Active Phase meal plans, 92–93
    hunger and, 84
    low-GI fruit for morning, 92
    never eat sweets, 139
    nuts for, 92–93, 179–180, 201
social support, 165–166
soluble fiber, 53–54
soups, 96–97
South Beach diet, 9, 125
sparkling waters
    club soda, 77, 192
    mineral water, 192
    seltzer water, 77, 192
    tonic water, 192–193
spices, 94, 193
spinach, 54, 82, 93, 191, 193
Splenda®, 61, 62
standard American diet (SAD)
    calories from sugar, 37–38
    carbohydrates and, 40–42
    fast and fried foods, 36–37
    low-fat diets and, 39–40
    overview of obesity contribution, 35–37
starch
    digestion of, 44
    on GI, 45
    glucose and, 44
    glycogen and, 44–46
    rapidly available, 45

refined, 45
resistant, 45
slowly available, 45
starving, 91, 184–185
　adaptive thermogenesis for, 126
　avoiding in Active Phase, 89
　goals and, 68
　inhibitory control and, 179–180
　Thinsulin Program prohibiting, 15,
　　100, 186
Statobex®, 213
staying on track
　in Active Phase, 19
　adherence level, 158–159
　boosting knowledge, 159–161
　mentorship, 166
　MI for, 161–165
　overview, 157–158
　social support, 165–166
stevia, 61
stigma, 207
stomach, 27 (fig.), 225
strawberries, 79, 115
stress, 67
　blood glucose and, 28
　inhibitory control and, 179
　weight gain and, 121
sucralose, 60–61
sucrose, 44, 55, 57, 61
suction-assisted liposuction (SAL),
　229
sugar, 27 (fig.), 31 (fig.), 33 (fig.),
　126
　as addictive, 58–60
　artificial sweeteners and, 62–64
　beverages, 57
　calories in SAD, 37–38
　cleansing system of, 178–179
　cravings, 70, 168, 185–186
　sugary drinks, 77, 140

UN and WHO recommendations,
　38
　weight gain and, 183
　See also sucrose; sweets
Sugar Twin®, 61
Sunett®, 60
Suprenza®, 212
Sweet One®, 60
SweetLeaf®, 61
Sweet'N Low®, 61
sweets, 112, 115
　in Active Phase food groups,
　　76–78
　beverages, 76–77
　cravings, 63, 139
　desserts, 68, 77–78, 123–124
　never as snack, 139
　in Passive Phase carbohydrates,
　　138–140
　sauces and condiments, 78
swimming, 149
sympathetic nervous system, 213
sympathy, 162

teaching, 160–161
Tecott, Laurence, 214
TEE. *See* total energy expenditure
Tenuate®, 213
Tenuate Dospan®, 213
Tepanil®, 213
Thinsulin Program
　addressing root of problem, 6
　alcohol and, 189–190
　Atkins and Paleo diets compared
　　to, 190–191
　biopsychosocial approach, 104,
　　106, 169, 183
　choices with, 70
　creation of, xx
　diabetes and, 203–204

Thinsulin Program *(continued)*
    Facebook page, 160
    for fighting obesity epidemic,
        187
    grouping foods, 63–64
    heart disease and, 204
    mental illness and, 205
    mind-body connection, 9
    as new beginning, 183–188
    night eating and, 200–201
    night workers on, 201–202
    paradigm shift, 187–188
    planning, 17
    pregnancy and, 204–205
    principles, 14, 158
    as realistic, 74
    results, 9–10
    starving prohibited, 15, 100, 186
    success stories, 5–9, 7 (photo),
        40, 41 (photo), 42, 69 (photo),
        70–71, 74, 75 (photo), 76, 112,
        113 (photo), 114, 122–124, 173,
        174 (photo), 175, 183–186,
        196–198, 199 (photo), 200
    teaching, 160–161
    understanding and motivation, 157
    vegetarians on, 195–196
    See also Active Phase; Active
        Phase, exercise; Active Phase,
        food groups; Active Phase, meal
        plans; Active Phase, milestones;
        Passive Phase; Passive Phase,
        carbohydrates and; Passive
        Phase, exercise; Passive Phase,
        milestones; Passive Phase,
        weight-loss-plateau and;
        specific topics
thyroid extract, 212
time discounting
    food cravings and, 180–182

science, 180
solution, 181–182
tofu, 84–87, 94
tomatoes, 82, 95, 96
tonic water, 192–193
TOS. *See* The Obesity Society
total energy expenditure (TEE), 130
triglycerides, 55, 57–59, 131
Truvia®, 61
tummy tuck, 230
turkey, 84, 88, 94, 115, 195

UN. *See* United Nations
unconscious neurobehavioral
        processes, 177, 179, 181
United Nations (UN), 38
University of Texas Health Science
        Center, 63
USDA, 38, 105

vagus nerve, 219
vascular dementia, 29–30
vegetables, 115
    191, 82
    in Active Phase food groups,
        81–84
    for dinners, 93–94
    fresh and raw, 83–84
    green leafy, 82, 84, 93, 149, 152,
        179–180, 204
    for lunches, 93–94
    in Passive Phase carbohydrates,
        137–138
    preparing, 193–194
    roots, tubers, kernels, 83–84
    See also specific vegetables
vegetarians
    ovo- and lacto-, 195
    on Thinsulin Program, 195–196
veggie burgers, 81, 196–197

Victoza®, 211
vitamins, 86, 212, 226
Vivus Inc., 217

walking, 101, 116
watermelon, 138
weighing in, 8
   for accountability, 164–165
   in Passive Phase, 19, 142, 144–145,
      153, 173
   as self-monitoring, 172–173
   weekly, 173
   with Weight Watchers®, 204
weight control, 67, 74, 97, 163,
   172, 205
weight gain
   antipsychotic medications and,
      xvi–xvii
   minimizing in Passive Phase,
      147
   punishment-reward-guilt
      cycle, 68
   stress and, 121
   sugar and, 183
weight management, 108
   insulin and, 30–32, 31 (fig.),
      33 (fig.)
   See also staying on track
Weight Watchers®, 125, 184–186,
   204
weight loss
   during Active Phase, 170
   activity and caloric intake
      emphasis, xvii–xviii
   behavioral therapy and, 169
   biology of, 107–108
   changing thinking, xix–xx
   cognitive distortions about, 109
   desire for, 110
   dual method for, xviii–xx

goals, 68–70
   insulin and, xiii, xviii, 183
   motivation for, 14–15, 122, 158
   New Year's resolutions, 122
   programs and products, 4–5
   psychiatry and, xv
   realistic expectations, 175–176
weight loss, journey of
   changing thinking, 21–22
   fishing in, 186
   motivations, 14–15
   overcoming myths, 14–22
   overview, 11–12
   success story, 13 (photo), 14
   ups and downs, 159
   willingness to change, 15
weight-loss plateau, xx, 8, 40,
   128 (fig.), 129 (fig.)
   overcoming, 114, 118
   See also Passive Phase,
      weight-loss-plateau and
weight-loss surgeries
   bariatric surgery, 224–227
   body contouring, 230–231
   candidates for, 228–229
   for combination restriction and
      malabsorption, 227–228
   costs, 228
   liposuction, 229–230
   for malabsorption, 226–227
   outcomes, 228–229
   overview, 223
   for restriction, 225–226
Wellbutrin®, 218
Wendy's, 106
wheat, 81–82, 136, 204
Wheat Belly (Davis), 80–81
WHO. *See* World Health
   Organization
whole foods, 45, 79

Wildwood products, 195
willpower, 177, 207–208, 220
wine belly, 81, 189
WIN-Nguyen diet, xvii–xviii
World Health Organization
    (WHO), 38, 61
World Journal of Surgery, 227

Xenical®, 211

yams, 82
yoga, 101–102, 148

Zumba, 101–102
Zyban®, 208, 218